# Cancer.
# Oh, Crap.

John J Powers III

*ISBN: 978-0-9892755-0-7 (Kindle)*
*ISBN: 978-0-9892755-1-4 (sc)*
*ISBN: 978-0-9892755-2-1 (ePub)*

*For Terry, the love of my life.*
*Don't unbuckle that seat belt just yet...*

# Foreword

Cancer Medicine.

I have been asked many times why I chose to go into this field. My original reason was always the same: a complex field which is constantly evolving and one where the docs are still the underdogs to the disease. The Rocky Balboa of medicine.

However as time has gone by, my perspective has changed a bit. While research is continuously reshaping our treatment options, it is only, after all, science, we can expect progress over time. Much more awe-inspiring is the power of the human spirit when confronted with a seemingly insurmountable obstacle.

Cancer is a disease that removes all of our social defenses. It strips us to our most basic form, and refocuses attention on our most basic instinct, survival. The privilege oncologists have to guide patients through this process is unlike any other that I have seen or heard described. The intimate connection as patient and doctor strive and push for a common goal, is the most rewarding aspect of this field. I see the will of my patients, their tenacity, their hope and their fear as my daily inspiration.

Hope and fear. This is the ying and yang of oncology.

While fear is always the initial emotion anyone experiences with a diagnosis of cancer, there is no doubt that hope is the strongest feeling they have throughout their ordeal. Hope is the fuel that burns at the core of all oncology patients, strong and steady.

Take this book and use it to learn, share, and overcome. Learn how to avoid common problems, what questions to ask, and when to seek help. Share your fears, concerns, joys, and love with those around you. Overcome fear by embracing hope, and trusting those who care for you.

Cancer fights can be long, draining events. It can't however, rob you of your hope or your smile.

As one of my favorite patients said to me:

*"No one fights alone."*

**Frank Rodriguez, M.D.**

# Acknowledgments

Special thanks to Frank Rodriguez, M.D., Florida Cancer Specialists, John J Green, D.O., the Angels of 2-West, Lee Memorial Health System, the Regional Cancer Center, H. Lee Moffitt Cancer Center and Research Institute, and each of the talented and dedicated managers, staff, nurses, doctors and employees therein. I am forever grateful to have somehow been fortunate enough to have been in your care. Saving a life may be routine for all of you, but for me it was certainly a new experience.

This book is a work of creative non-fiction, as the author is not 100% certain of every detail. Written notes made while medicated may not be entirely accurate. Those notes and other documents were used to reconstruct many events. Every effort was made to provide the actual truth. Any error, omission or misstatement of fact is purely unintentional.

# Introduction

This book was written to serve various audiences and points of view.

The Cancer Patient

You should know that there is help and there is hope. You should also know that, in addition to your medical status, your attitude and demeanor are cues your caregivers will use to make judgments concerning your well-being. As Terry reminded me often, "Nobody likes a whiner." Give your caregiver a break, and be sure to say "Thank you."

The Medical Professional

You may not be used to hearing our point of view because you are too busy trying to save our lives. We have put our trust in you, and our future is in your hands. Communicate. Tell the truth without regard to our feelings. While you are making notes when standing over us at bedside, we are paying careful attention to your body language and facial expressions. We already know that you care. We know when you are concerned, and we know when you are not willing to share the whole truth. We know when you are bored and would rather be somewhere else, and when you are in a rush to leave. We can sense that you are afraid or unsure. We can also sense competence, confidence and empathy.

The Blood Donor

The unsung hero. Without your charity and kindness, many of us would not be alive today. Your gift matters to someone every day. On behalf of cancer patients and blood donation recipients everywhere; thank you from the bottom of our hearts.

Everybody Else

We all know someone affected by cancer. Try to see things from their perspective, but understand that they do not expect, nor want, your pity. To acknowledge that cancer is present will be enough. To offer transportation to or from a medical appointment, or to offer help with a household chore would certainly be gratefully accepted and much appreciated. One last request: Please do not talk to others about us in the third person when we are in the same room. We're here, we're alive, and we'd like to participate.

# Prologue

It is a glorious Sunday around noon in mid-October. The sun is streaming in through the sliding glass doors, silently massaging my back as I sit at the kitchen table eating a sandwich while navigating the large weekend newspaper. A family of ducks at lake's edge just outside my door quacks out an opera only they know the lyrics to, and there is a large snow-white egret looking for his lunch. My northern friends refer to this place as 'God's Waiting Room', while the automobile license tags sport oversized oranges and proclaim this to be the 'Sunshine State'.

After lunch I headed for the living room to watch a game on television. It's been a long time since I've felt this well and Terry seems pleased that the worst appears to be over. She has put her recent memories into an imaginary drawer labeled *"History – let's hope the worst has passed."*

Not five minutes later, an all too familiar feeling washes over me and I instinctively know what the next few hours will bring; not because I'm smart, but rather because we've been through this before. A quick swipe over my forehead with the temporal artery scanner reveals an elevated temperature of 102.9°. I try to head this fever off at the pass by swallowing a few Tylenol pills. Ten minutes later my temperature is somewhere north of 103° and I confirm this finding with an oral thermometer. My system is obviously trying to fight off an infection of some kind.

Terry is already packing my overnight bag for a trip to the emergency room. A temperature of 101.5° is considered life-threatening for me because my immune system is impaired. There is no point in calling my oncologist's answering service because we know the drill. Get to the emergency room ASAP. As we leave the house my thermometer displays 104° and I know we're in trouble again. . .

# Chapter 1

Cancer. There, I said it. My name is John and I have cancer.

This is my story; the story of my journey with cancer. I am a 56-year-old male who woke up one day and learned that I had blood cancer. Acute Myelogenous Leukemia (AML) to be exact. This disease is also known as Acute Myeloid Leukemia, Acute Myelolytic Leukemia, Acute Myeloblastic Leukemia, Acute Granulocytic Leukemia and Acute Nonlymphocytic Leukemia.

I'll try not to bore you to tears, or waste your time with unnecessary medical terminology or too much science. That said, there are some basic definitions that you should be familiar with so you may understand what is happening while treatments are given and problems arise. You'll see these terms constantly. Please bear with me; I'll keep it short and as painless as possible.

Leukemia is the general term for some different types of blood cancer. AML is one of four main types of leukemia.

### Red Cells[1]

Red cells make up 40-45% of the blood. They are filled with hemoglobin, the protein that picks up oxygen in the lungs and delivers it to cells all around the body.

### Platelets[1]

Platelets are small cell fragments, one-tenth the size of red cells, which help stop bleeding at the site of an injury in the body. For example, when a person gets a cut, the vessels that carry blood are torn open. Platelets stick to the torn surface of the vessel, clump together and plug up the bleeding site. Later, a firm clot forms. The vessel wall then heals at the site of the clot and returns to its normal state.

### White Cells[1]

Unlike red cells and platelets, the white cells leave the blood and enter the tissues, where they can ingest invading organisms and help combat infection. There are two major types of white cells: germ-eating cells (neutrophils and monocytes) and lymphocytes.

### Marrow[1]

Marrow is a spongy tissue where blood cell development takes place. It occupies the central

---

[1] From The Leukemia & Lymphoma Society

cavity of bones. In newborns, all bones have active marrow. By the time a person reaches young adulthood, the bones of the hands, feet, arms and legs no longer have functioning marrow. The back bones (vertebrae), hip and shoulder bones, ribs, breastbone and skull contain marrow that makes blood cells in adults. Blood passes through the marrow and picks up formed red and white cells and platelets for circulation.

Complete Blood Count (CBC)[1]

Blood is drawn often to measure the levels of blood components for comparison to normal.

Bone Marrow Biopsy[1]

Biopsies are taken on a regular basis to examine cells withdrawn from marrow within a bone to detect abnormalities and to compare with biopsies performed at an earlier date (staging).

Now that we've covered the educational portion of this odyssey, let's get on with the story. There is more to discover, but I'll sprinkle it in as we go.

# Chapter 2

*The Beginning*

Thursday, March 31, 2011

This journey began with a visit to my physician, Dr. John Green. I made an appointment because I've had a headache for three or four weeks and have been taking Motrin by the handful. I've found that Motrin is about the only thing that will kill these headaches quickly. I've also been short of breath. I looked it up on the internet and found this is called dyspnea. I'm not talking about running a mile and breathing heavily. I mean that I walked up one flight of stairs behind my 83-year-old mother and had to stop at the top to catch my breath while she skittered off to fetch herself a glass of wine. This might not raise a red flag for some of you, but Mom was considering heart surgery at the time to open a main artery for better circulation. Aortic stenosis, I think she called it.

My primary physician Dr. Green is a very smart and efficient doctor, with a staff to match. I called for an appointment to discover the cause of this shortness of breath and ongoing headache and I got it for the same day. No muss, no fuss, didn't have to whine or fabricate symptoms; I just called and was given the appointment. Hopefully, this was just the first of many miracles in store for me.

After a quick examination later that day, Dr. Green said that I looked anemic and ordered blood tests to get some additional information. I stopped on the way home and had my blood drawn as ordered. The Lee Memorial Health System outpatient blood draw center is the greatest concept since banks began to put in drive-through service. Walk in, present your insurance card and identification, and have your blood drawn. No waiting. No year-old magazines. No elevator music. Just step this way, John, and I'll take some blood. Thank you very much. You just can't find service like this anymore. This operation is efficient, courteous and friendly. Another miracle already; it feels like I'm on a roll today.

8:00 p.m. and Dr. Green calls my home phone to leave a message that I should call him first thing tomorrow. Are you kidding? A doctor is calling the house? After hours? I feel blessed. At least until the recording says "*We* have a problem." By "*We*" I'm pretty sure he means "*me*." OK, I'll call back tomorrow, first thing in the morning.

Friday, April 1, 2011

That day stuck in my mind because it was April Fools' Day. I was on my way to a jobsite and my cell phone rang. It was early, too early for me to have called Dr. Green, but there he was, on my phone very early on a Friday morning. I dislike phones and don't usually answer mine while driving, but the caller ID got my attention. I pulled my truck out of traffic over to the curb, and answered the call.

Dr. Green related that my blood counts are very, very low. We needed to do something about it right away. When I explained that my Dad had low levels of B12 and maybe I've inherited the same deficiency, he doesn't buy it. When I said that I probably don't get enough exercise or eat enough vegetables, and that I'll mend my ways, he still doesn't buy it. He thinks "*We*" have a serious problem, and that I have not listened to what he has said.

The good doctor explained that I needed a referral and, when arranged, someone on his staff would call me back. A few short minutes later, Elaine called to inform me that I have an appointment for Monday morning, 9:00 a.m. at Florida Cancer Specialists. "Excuse me; you have made a terrible mistake. This is *John* Powers you're speaking with."

"Mr. Powers, you need this appointment," she told me.

Florida *CANCER* Specialists? Oh, crap, this can't be good. I hope my friends were wrong when they called Florida 'God's Waiting Room'.

# Chapter 3

Monday, April 4<sup>th</sup>

First thing in the morning I received a telephone call at home. A young woman's voice from Florida Cancer Specialists explained, "Sorry, but we don't see new patients on Mondays."

For one of the few times that I can recall, I became assertive and replied that this was not acceptable. I didn't schedule the appointment; you did, after all. The newly assertive me eventually prevailed and was told to come on in and they would figure something out. I'm thinking maybe this assertive behavior will come in handy at other times as well.

Arriving at Florida Cancer Specialists (FCS), the first order of business for my wife Terry and I is money, of course. Money is the engine that makes the world go 'round. Financial counseling in the business office included an explanation of our health insurance plan benefits. We discover what amount my co-payments will be for each visit, what my annual deductible and out-of-pocket maximums will be, and what other expenses we should expect. None of this news sounds good, and it's sure to end up costing a fortune that we just don't have. Terry maintains our health insurance through her employer, and we are grateful that this insurance is in place.

I decided right then and there that I will try not to dwell on the financial aspects of cancer. I will pay all that I am able, and we will put together the other financial puzzle pieces as we go. I recently sold my Harley-Davidson motorcycle and wonder if the cash might come in handy soon. I am reminded of the last time I sold a motorcycle. It was during 1976, and the cash raised from the sale was used to buy and install a bay window. Gee, priorities sure have a habit of getting in the way of my life.

After leaving the business office in a mild state of shock, we were sent back to the crowded waiting area. The waiting room here is scary. There are many people here with barely a few strands of hair on their heads. Some are holding oxygen tanks and others have various kinds of carrying cases and fanny packs with tubes sticking out and going to who knows where. Many wear a mask that covers their mouth and nose to prevent airborne infection. Aluminum rolling walkers and uncomfortable-looking wheelchairs are well represented. CNN is tuned in, but silent on the wall-mounted plasma television, and year-old National Geographic magazines are displayed on the small wooden end tables. I swear I can see apparitions floating eerily a few feet above the floor. They are wearing flowing white robes; their hairless skulls are wrapped in kerchiefs or bandanas of some kind, and each one carries either an oxygen tank or fanny pack that contains some kind of medical apparatus. They are strangely reminiscent of the group I am now seated among.

I'm beginning to think I might have a really serious problem on my hands.

# Chapter 4

Soon, I am escorted to the laboratory area to have blood drawn for CBCs. I'm beginning to develop an aversion to needles already. I just had blood drawn last Friday; why again so soon? Had I known how many times this would happen over the next few months I would have fainted on the spot. There is so much I don't know about all of this, and I made a mental note to do more research. A *lot* more research.

After the blood draw, we had a short wait in a tiny exam room. The room was outfitted with a couple of chairs and an examination table with a giant roll of tan paper standing by for a new patient. A networked desktop computer station sat on a small desk.

Soon, I met Dr. Francisco (Frank) Rodriguez for the very first time. I have never met an oncologist before today and hoped that I never would, except on a golf course. He is 35 or 40-ish, and according to Terry, a very handsome man. He looked ordinary to me as he shook my hand and introduced himself. Dr. Rodriguez and I will have a very close relationship for many months, and perhaps years, to come.

Dr. Rodriguez explained that my CBC test results indicate the need to perform a bone marrow biopsy. I thought to myself, "OK, let's make an appointment for sometime during the next few weeks or maybe next month." No such luck. Dr. Rodriguez said, "Unbuckle your belt, lower your pants some, hop up and lie face down on the examining table. Let's get this done." Oh, great. This is not something I had planned as one of today's activities.

Next, Dr. Rodriguez explained to me that, after a local anesthetic, a rather large, hollow needle-like instrument (read: drill bit) will be inserted into my hipbone from the rear until passing through the bone and reaching into the marrow. This apparatus will then collect a marrow sample to be used for laboratory inspection and analysis.

The insertion of the drill bit, I mean needle, didn't bother me at all until I could clearly hear a crunching sound as it passed through my hip bone on its way to the marrow. Repeated attempts to gently retract the bit that had just collected a marrow sample are not successful. Dr. Rodriguez finally pulled so hard on the darn thing that I was lifted right up off of the table and dropped back down more than once. I quickly realized that Dr. Rodriguez is a lot stronger than he appears to be.

No matter what the future results of this biopsy might indicate, I was told that I needed to receive a blood transfusion ASAP.

# Chapter 5

Tuesday, April 5, 2011

Today I arrived at the Regional Cancer Center building for an early morning appointment to get my first blood transfusion. I think of this as getting my fluids topped off.

The office park where the Regional Cancer Center is located is commonly referred to as The Sanctuary. There are a host of medical offices, outpatient facilities, radiology services, a transfusion center, chemotherapy services and radiation therapy offices, and of course, a few restaurants. Everything a cancer patient might need, all in a remarkably convenient proximity. Score one for urban planning.

Apparently my hemoglobin measurement of 5 is quite low and I require a blood transfusion. I'm told a hemoglobin level of 15 is normal for someone my size and age, and that I will need the addition of two units of blood. Feeling tired and rundown? Go get some new blood; it works wonders. I've donated blood in the past but have never been on the receiving end until now.

After filling out a mound of paperwork at the registration desk, the receptionist asked what I'd like to have for lunch. I thought to myself that the poor woman was fighting the bell curve of senility, and didn't realize that it was only about 8:00 a.m. Possessing full control of my own faculties, I replied that I was only here for some blood and would be gone long before lunchtime. "No dear," she stated with a look of empathy, "you'll certainly still be here at lunchtime, would you like to order a meal?" Rather than argue with her, I chose a deli sandwich and bottled water from the menu. She then fitted an identification bracelet onto my wrist and asked me to have a seat while I waited to be transfused for the very first time.

After a brief wait, I was brought by a nurse into a large, open area filled with what appeared to be first class cabin leather reclining chairs in orderly rows of perhaps six across. Adjacent to each chair was a metal stand with an attached electronic pump used for intravenous (IV) therapy. There must be ten or twelve rows of these stations stretching out some eighty feet to the far wall and wrapped around a countertop where nurses are busy at computer stations and telephones. There are perhaps a half dozen other patients already here with long, clear tubes filled with blood, platelets or other liquids hooked up to them. I tried not to look, but couldn't seem to help myself. I compared this urge to look around me as the same urge others might have when passing the scene of a car crash.

The entire space is well lighted, bright and airy, with large windows overlooking the bordering green foliage. The view from up here on the second floor is soothing and is in stark contrast to the business at hand within these four walls.

I was introduced to a pleasant nurse who guided me to an empty station. Because I was a newbie, she explained very slowly and carefully the events that were to follow. I swallowed two Tylenol pills with the help of a few sips from a provided bottle of water while she gently planted a needle into a vein in my wrist. I didn't feel a thing; she's done this before and I felt instantly at ease.

Next, a clear plastic bag containing a unit of dark red blood was delivered to my station by another nurse. I wonder why they refer to these as 'units' as opposed to a volume measurement like a pint or quart or even liters. Perhaps there is no standard amount.

In unison, the two nurses announced and repeated my name, medical record number, date of birth, blood type, expiration date and the fact that this unit of blood is irradiated. Units of blood and blood products are irradiated to eliminate impurities.

I wondered if this irradiated blood flowing through my veins would make me glow in the dark. . .

The headache I had lived with for what seemed like months melted away soon after the first unit of blood was transfused. The actions of the morning were repeated for the second unit as my lunch was delivered and placed on a hide-away tray attached to my recliner. Maybe these seats did come from first class.

I was sent back to the waiting area shortly after receiving the second unit of blood. A short waiting period was required to be sure I experienced no adverse reactions. Five and one-half hours had ticked away since my early arrival. I recalled the lunch conversation from earlier, and thanked the receptionist as she wished me good luck. I also silently gave thanks to those who routinely donate blood and blood products. I vowed to join these people and make routine donations should I ever get through this.

I skipped the elevator ride and took the stairs two at a time down to the main lobby. Surely nobody with any kind of cancer could do this, I foolishly thought to myself.

# Chapter 6

*The Diagnosis*

Wednesday, April 6, 2011

I arrived at the hospital for an abdominal ultrasound. The ultrasound will measure and image my stomach, gallbladder, spleen, kidneys, lungs and liver to discover any existing anomalies. The resulting images may also be used as a baseline comparison as we move forward with treatments.

Perhaps they will also discover a use for these images as a model reference to extol the benefits of clean and healthy living. After all, my body is my temple.

This daydream ended abruptly as I walked right into a closed glass door.

Friday April 8, 2011

A few days later we are back with Dr. Rodriguez to hear the results of my bone marrow biopsy. Results are not 100% conclusive, but I certainly have a population of immature and malformed stem cells called blasts. Terry said, "Gee, what a surprise; immature? Who would have guessed?" Apparently, some of my bone marrow cells don't mature as designed. These resulting blast cells will continue to build up, and will eventually prevent any normal blood cell production.

Diagnosis: We are somewhere between MDS (Myelodysplastic Syndrome; think Robin Roberts from *Good Morning America*) and AML (Acute Myelogenous Leukemia). Neither is a good thing; both dictate the necessity of immediate treatment. I feel screwed and actually wondered briefly if anybody else has ever had this same diagnosis before me, because I sure feel alone right now.

After a lengthy discussion of treatment options with Dr. Rodriguez, we elect to treat this cancer aggressively. Aggressively, in this case, means four to five weeks of inpatient chemotherapy treatment. I will receive a '7+3' regimen, which translates to a chemical cocktail of cytarabine each day for seven days and a booster of idarubicin on each of the first three days. This will be followed by a recovery period of approximately three weeks. The treatment is designed to kill all but the base stem cells and, if successful, it will be thirty days and I'm done.

Before we begin treatment, however, Dr. Rodriguez thinks I should get a second opinion; his office will make arrangements and will advise me later today concerning the particulars. The H. Lee Moffit Cancer Center in Tampa may recommend that I consider a bone marrow transplant as a treatment option.

# Chapter 7

Later the same day, I received a phone call from an administrator at the Moffit Center in Tampa. She informed me that Moffit was 'out of network' for my health insurance plan. I responded that this was acceptable and I would pay the 20%, or whatever the out of network percentage charge will actually be. To my chagrin, I was then told to "bring a check for $5,000 and have available an additional $5,000, readily accessible, just in case." Ouch.

When I picked myself up off of the floor, I asked, "Are you serious? This is a consultation that may last a few hours and you want upwards of $5,000 for an opinion *in addition* to any insurance benefit we may receive?" I was told that I understood correctly. I immediately said that I could not afford this, and I needed to call the insurance company to see if we might work something out.

Terry and I quickly realized that we will probably be bankrupt by the end of my treatments; whatever these treatments will turn out to be. I have heard before that cancer is only one piece of the puzzle, and the financial impact can seem more devastating than the disease. Naively, I thought that comprehensive insurance coverage would shield us from the misfortune and indignity that has befallen others in our situation. Wrong again.

We've been told that any costs not paid by the insurance company must be paid by us. I signed paperwork to that effect a few times already, but trusted that insurance purchased through a company employee plan would actually cover our medical expenses. Our financial responsibility after deductibles, co-pays and co-insurance amounts is apparently unlimited. Annual maximum out-of-pocket amounts are a mirage and are not to be believed when encountering certain out of network situations.

My initial plea for help from the insurance company was directed to answering machines that didn't seem to care. When I finally reached a real person, she seemed to care even less. My request for referral to somebody in the company who could help with my predicament was met with a polite, but firm, "Sorry, sir, we can't help you." A plea for help made to the Human

Resources department where Terry works resulted in a referral directly back to the insurance company. I was dizzy from all of the run-arounds I was getting.

I eventually surrendered to the red tape and elected to entrust my life to Dr. Rodriguez. I was already tired of dealing with insurance, administrators and business office personnel who just didn't seem to care. Why should they? It is my disease, my problem, my life. I had a lousy attitude already, and wondered how I could ever go through a cancer treatment regimen if I felt defeated before we even began.

I called the Moffit Center administrator and asked that she cancel the appointment because I could not afford to pay for it. I called Dr. Rodriguez and told him what happened with his referral and that I was ready to begin treatment.

I own and operate a small business that requires my availability to respond to emergencies 24/7. My treatment will make this availability impossible and may even put the very survival of this business in jeopardy.

Dr. Rodriguez wanted my hospital stay to begin immediately, but I negotiated with him to buy time to find a replacement to operate the business during my expected absence. I also needed to meet and speak with each of my customers to explain why I needed someone to fill in for me.

# Chapter 8

Sunday, April 10, 2011

The doorbell rang and I walked down the stairway to respond. We seldom had unannounced visitors, so I wondered which of our neighbors required assistance.

When the door was opened, I found a screaming baby in a car seat perched on the porch. I sure hoped that someone hadn't abandoned the child; Terry already had my infantile behavior to deal with.

This is an unexpected visit from my out-of-state son, John, and his family. The crying baby is my grandson John; now nearly seven months old. I will remember this week-long visit and cherish the memories for the rest of my life; however long that may turn out to be. I wrote a note to myself that day. It read: "This is the moment against which all others will be measured from this day forward."

Cancer. Oh, Crap.

Prior to my inpatient stay there was a lot to accomplish. My visiting son helped me to complete some outstanding business for my customers. Terry and I fawned endlessly over our grandson and enjoyed every moment. I had forgotten how much fun vomit and diarrhea could be when it belonged to someone else's child.

The week was full of surprises and gifts conceived in the kind hearts of my family. My son and his wife, Stacy, gathered family pictures and assembled them in a beautiful picture frame. The frame would be proudly displayed in my hospital room to remind me of what was at stake. Gifts of pajamas, slippers, pillow, tee shirts and written mementos were gratefully received. It seemed as though they thought of everything. I counted myself a lucky man to have family by my side as I embarked on this journey to parts unknown.

I also found time to perform research on my disease. Treatment issues, survival probability statistics and possible complications were studied and logged.

We'll talk more about survival probabilities later. The statistics are grim and indicate a very uncertain future.

# Chapter 9

Early in the morning of Monday, April 18<sup>th</sup>, Terry brought me and my large duffle bag to the hospital. The duffle bag was full of personal items Stacy and John purchased as gifts.

During the registration process, lots of intake forms and paperwork needed my attention and signatures. I usually read and re-read anything I am required to sign or initial, but the sheer volume of these forms was ridiculous. I eventually surrendered and signed everything they put in front of me with barely a glance. Hell, I may die during this treatment; why haggle over a few minor legalities that I signed under duress?

An identification bracelet was fitted to my wrist and we were escorted to 2-West, one of the two cancer floors in the hospital. Cancer used to be something that other, less fortunate people ended up with. I never gave cancer much thought, but there we were on the cancer floor and I really did not like it much. Bald people in standard hospital garb were being escorted down the hallways by their rolling IV stands with hanging bags of medicines on one arm and a nurse or family member on the other. Masks covered their noses and mouths. God, they looked awful and I was secretly glad not to have been them. Nurses seemed cheerful although I'm not sure why; there didn't seem to be anything to be cheerful about. Nursing aides carefully pushed small carts stuffed with paperwork and electronic blood pressure monitors. Uniformed clinicians reading information attached to clipboards darted from one room to the next, food service carts were being dragged along by their attendants, and an occasional doctor with a stethoscope necktie was seen scurrying about. Everyone seemed fully engaged in taking care of the business of cancer.

This was beginning to feel real, and for the first time the gravity of this whole situation started to weigh on me. I felt engulfed, like when the morning fog wrapped itself around the trees and clung to the lake behind my home. I didn't like the way I was feeling, and wondered bitterly what I did to deserve this fate. I guess I was far too preoccupied with making sure those around me were able to deal with the enormity of this, and assuring them that everything would be OK. I repeated those assurances often enough so that even I believed this whole affair was just a speed bump in the road of my life.

After introductions to my new family of nurses and aides, I settled into a room featuring a state-of-the-art hospital bed that seemed to have more controls than a small airplane. There was a private bathroom and shower that I immediately appreciated. I did not immediately appreciate the hospital gown so helpfully provided for me. I was certain that somehow this had been just a big mistake, and if they could see me wearing my own pajamas and tee shirts, everyone would realize I was the victim of a very cruel hoax. I expected to wake up any moment to discover this was just a dream. Denial is not just a river in Africa.

The remaining daylight hours were eaten up with a myriad of medical studies of their newest cancer patient. A blood draw, urine collection, blood pressure and heart rate monitoring, and a MUGA scan were all on the menu. A MUGA scan (multilayer acquisition scan) creates video images of the heart ventricles to check whether they are pumping blood properly.

# Chapter 10

The next day, there were more staff introductions, and a notable visit from someone in the psychology department.

First, a little background is in order. Most people in my small circle of friends enjoy a cocktail or two on occasion. I am no exception, and count myself as about average when measuring cocktail consumption against others in my peer group.

When I filled out the hospital entrance exam questionnaires, I truthfully answered all of their questions. This included the questions that assumed it was necessary to pry into one's drinking habits. Telling the truth was a huge mistake. Take it from me, and repeat this three times slowly; never, ever, ever, be even remotely accurate when describing the volume and frequency of your alcohol intake to a medical professional.

Now back to the wolf in sheep's clothing, I mean the shrink. He was a slight and frail-looking man named Edmund[2], who was in his late fifties or early sixties. His jet-black hair was in such disarray it must have been combed with a firecracker. His skin was wrinkled and translucent, and looked like it would crack if touched. Behind wire-rimmed eyeglasses, his beady gray eyes had a laser-like focus that seemed to penetrate my exterior clear to the bone. His lips were thin and tight, and when he began to speak, I swore I could see a lick of fire spitting from his tongue. Surprisingly, his voice was calm and gentle, but still ominously accusatory.

Edmund introduced himself, then immediately warned Terry and me that one who abused alcohol to my extent would no doubt be a troublesome patient. He suggested that I be detoxified and medicated before chemotherapy treatment, lest I go on a maniacal rampage when my lust for alcohol is not satiated. Those weren't his exact words, but those were the words we heard. We understood this to mean that treatment would be denied if I refused his pre-treatment suggestions.

Who did he think he was? He never met us, and knew nothing about me; only what I

---

[2] Not his real name

willingly divulged in the registration forms. Yet here he was, prepared to deny life-saving cancer treatment to someone who has just been torn apart by the news of having this horrible disease.

Terry vehemently protested Edmund's assessment and suggestions, and gave him a small piece of her mind. Terry let him know that if he continued down that road, his next move would be directly out the second floor window. I tried to tell Terry that Edmund was just doing his job, but she had heard enough. It was time for Eddie to hit the road.

We later learned from the nurses that they are trained to multiply by a factor of three any answer you willingly divulge concerning alcohol or drug intake. So apparently if you drink, you are a liar as well. Be forewarned so as not to endure this embarrassing treatment yourself.

Throughout the day I was transfused with blood products. Two units of blood and one unit of platelets were on today's menu. These products were all irradiated at a remote location and delivered by courier. Like my previous transfusions at the Sanctuary, nurses read the labels, compared numbers on the orders to my medical ID bracelet, and simultaneously announced the specifics. I appreciated their attention to detail and felt blessed to have such people caring for me. This was life or death; they have seen too much of the latter and wouldn't let a mistake on their part put runs on the scoreboard for the opposing team.

# Chapter 11

Rise and shine! It's all been a bad dream! From the spartan furnishings, drab wall hangings and window shades, it seemed I was in a cheap motel. I could even smell the aroma of strong coffee just outside of my closed door. I did, however, have a hazy memory of being disturbed every few hours to have my vitals taken by a CNA (Certified Nursing Assistant). My suspicions were quickly confirmed, as the room service waitress with the coffee is not a waitress at all, but rather an NSA (Nutrition Services Assistant). It turned out that the coffee was not for me anyway, because I was NPO.

NPO is an acronym for the Latin "nil per os," and means "nothing by mouth." To me, it is English and means "no coffee for you." I miss my coffee, and I may go on a rampage if I don't get some soon. Maybe Eddie was on the right track…

I was NPO because apparently I was prepping for surgery. Surgery? Excuse me; I don't recall signing up for any surgeries. My protests were ignored and I was ordered out of my comfy pajamas and tee shirt and into a hospital gown. I feigned insult and modesty, but nobody seemed to care. They were sterile garments and were the required clothing for a trip to the operating suite where I would receive a dual, two-chamber mediport. The mediport implant would be surgically placed in the upper portion of my right chest and have a delivery system catheter originating from within the port, up my chest, over my collarbone and directly into my jugular vein. I was informed that this implant would be a part of me for a long, long time.

The purpose of a mediport is to allow all intravenous medicines and chemotherapy drugs to be delivered directly to the bloodstream. There would be no need to make another needle puncture in an arm or wrist vein in order to receive medicines and fluids. I guess that after puncturing your veins every few hours for one reason or another day after day, at some point the vein may not be structurally sound enough to continue.

I took a quick shower, brushed my teeth and shaved my face. Little did I realize, soon there wouldn't be a need to shave because of hair loss, a shower would be a luxury because I'd be tied up to chemo and IV equipment by gobs of tubing, and my gums and mouth would bleed so easily that it would be difficult, and even painful to brush my teeth.

I was delivered to the OR on a transport gurney. The OR nurses made quick work of preparation that included vitals measurements, the usual mound of paperwork and a chest X-ray. I was given a sedative of what I refer to as 'goofy juice'. I liked goofy juice because it worked quickly and allowed no time to think or worry about what was to happen next.

The next thing I knew, I was waking up in the recovery room. I found a two to three-inch long horizontal sewn-up incision and a rather large lump under the skin on my chest. A catheter that felt like a small straw travelled up and away from the lump, and then over the collarbone and stitched into place. For a brief moment I wondered what kind of mind would dream up a device like that.

I made the trip back to my new home on 2-West on another transport gurney. Terry later told me that, upon my return, I jumped up from the transport bed and exclaimed, "I'm cured!"

I can neither confirm nor deny that actually happened, but Terry would never lie. Not even when you need to hear just a slightly different version of the truth. I wrote off my odd behavior to the goofy juice. Did I mention that I like goofy juice?

It was a very long day and I drifted off to sleep quickly. Every few hours I woke up to a CNA scheduled to retrieve my vitals, but otherwise the night passed uneventfully.

Morning arrived right on time and a friendly NSA appeared with the 'Chef's Special' breakfast and a paper cup filled just past the halfway mark with lukewarm coffee. The Chef's Special was the meal served when nothing else was ordered.

I made a mental note to fill out my menu order before the deadline time each day so the Chef's Special wouldn't become my sole source of nutrition. I'm sure the meals are nutritiously correct, but based on the looks, temperature and taste; I'd prefer a "chicken or pasta?" meal served by a flight attendant.

# Chapter 12

*Chemo begins*

Upon return from an early morning walk around 2-West, I noticed three signs attached to the wall outside my door that I didn't recall seeing before. One declared the inhabitant (me) "neutropenic" while the others said "chemotherapy precautions" and "bleeding risk, oral thermometers only." Oh-oh, this can't be good. The bathroom wall was also wearing a sign that read "Chemotherapy, be sure to flush twice." I was going to add 'because it's a long way to the cafeteria', but thought that a bit sophomoric.

Neutropenic means that I don't have enough neutrophils. A neutrophil is one type of white blood cell that finds and kills bacteria in your body. Chemotherapy can cause bone marrow to make fewer neutrophils, which will leave one vulnerable to infection because of this lowered defense capability. Precautions to avoid bacteria and infection, such as wearing a mask and constant hand-washing must be observed.

Laurie Lee, a friend of ours, visited the morning of my first chemo infusion. She is a nurse who was working on another floor, and had taken time at the tail end of her twelve-hour night shift to stop by. Laurie continued to visit throughout all of my inpatient stays, which spanned a period of seven months. Imagine the effort required to continue doing that after working a busy shift for more than twelve hours! Her husband John, a golf buddy of mine, dropped in often to offer his support as well. I'm not sure what we did to be blessed with friends like this, but I was, and remain, extremely grateful.

Halfway through the morning, a nurse showed up to access my mediport. To do this, she would take an inch-long needle with a small yellow tubing manifold attached, and force the needle through my skin into the titanium reservoir cup that is the port. My mediport is a dual, and has two of these cups. The needle would continue to be forced in until the flat manifold was seated flush to my skin. I would be lying if I told you this was painless. To top it off, because my mediport was a dual, the procedure had to be done twice.

The nurses must have been trained by vampires, judging by the pleasure they seemed to derive from that chore. After completion there was access directly to my bloodstream via the jugular. I wondered how many tubes were expected to be delivering liquid chemicals and other fluids into me. I saw two needles; each sporting a 'Y' tubing connector. My math skills were sharp enough to know that we now had four separate routes into my port and I wondered if they would piggyback some more of these 'Y' connectors to increase my productivity.

The nurse explained that my port must be flushed before and after any fluids are introduced. She took the plug out of one of the tubes and then attached the tube to a small syringe filled with heparin. Heparin is a blood thinner used to prevent clots from forming on the inside of the tubing or port. The plunger was depressed, and before I ever saw fluid flowing, I could taste it. That seemed really strange to me, but I was assured that it was considered normal. Four tubes of blood were extracted through the newly-cleansed port for CBC testing, and then the heparin flush was repeated.

Soon, the nurse returned with an IV stand. The stand was a six-foot tall chromed-metal contraption with open-ended eyelet fixture arms welded to a thick center post. The center post was seated into and attached to a four-legged base with round rolling casters. Plastic IV containers would hang from the eyelet fixture hooks before being attached to the recipient by clear plastic tubing.

Attached to the stand was a vice-like fixture that was in turn securing a device that would control the flow of chemicals as they were fed into my port. The electronic device had a membrane keyboard, LED display and a small door that opened to reveal a miniature pump into which the incoming fluids would be fed and their flow regulated. This IV pump was truly a modern electro-mechanical device that I was sure to have some fun with. Electronics, machinery and computers have always fascinated me, and I couldn't wait to find out how the controls on this pump operated.

A clear bag of saline was hung from one of the hooks on the IV stand, and the first of the hundreds of tubes I would see during the next month was installed. Tubing was first attached to the saline bag, and then to one of the clear 'Y' tubes protruding from the manifold on my port.

A new nurse appeared with an additional clear bag filled with fluid. The skull and crossbones on the label told me all I needed to know, but the nurse felt compelled to explain. It is cytarabine, and it is dangerous. It is the 'chemo' in chemotherapy. Don't spill it on yourself because it will burn. Burn? Are you kidding me? If it will burn your skin why the heck would you possibly consider putting this chemical directly into my bloodstream? I was instantly skeptical of this whole plan and wondered if I would live to see tomorrow.

As I tried to calm myself, the bag containing this powerful chemical was hung from the IV stand and attached to the IV pump with a clear tube. Another tube was attached to the pump and then to my port. Before the pump was started, a few things needed to occur. First, a steroid drop was put into each of my eyes. Next up was a handwriting test where I was instructed to provide my signature. This was a sample reference to which an après-chemo signature would be compared. I hoped that I still remembered my name when that time came.

I learned that signature comparisons could tell a story of vital importance to a medical professional. My mental state would be evaluated for changes should my signature differ in certain ways when compared to the sample. A signature difference may indicate that chemo has affected my mental processes.

Next came a small cup that looked like it was stolen from my dentist's office; you know, the small beige crinkly-sided paper cup used to rinse and spit? The cup was loaded with the preventives Decadron, Zofran and Tylenol.

Decadron (dexamathasone) is a cortical steroid that relieves inflammation-caused pain I didn't yet have; Zofran (ondansetron HCl) is used to prevent or to lessen the nausea I was starting to feel after seeing all that medicine, and I was pretty sure the Tylenol was for the nurse, in case I whined too much about having to take all of the other pills.

Having swallowed the required appetizers, we continued on to the main course of chemo. As the IV pump was being programmed to provide the appropriate flow of the clear liquid, I wondered if I would ever be the same from that moment in time forward. I'd be lying if I said I had a good feeling about any of this, and suddenly wondered what God had planned for me.

God and I have a two-part deal that I made a while back and I thought He may want to collect soon. Not being one to renege on a deal, I silently told Him that I was fully prepared to pay up anytime He saw fit. As if I was calling the shots.

Ninety minutes later, the clear bag that used to be full of cytarabine was shriveled up like the old gal in the room next door. The IV pump was emitting an irritating *beep-beep, beep-beeep, beep-beeep*. Listening to the racket that thing was making, I thought that nurses, doctors and maybe the board of directors would be hustling towards my room. As I listened carefully for the footsteps of my rescue party, I heard faint choruses of other machines *beep-beeeping* as they all were competing for somebody's attention. Being new to all this, I didn't dare try to silence this alarm, for fear that over my grave they would all be whispering, "If only he let the alarm go on he'd probably still be with us." I'm sure I only imagined someone else saying, "Serves the bastard right."

After what seemed an eternity, my nurse arrived and silenced the alarm. She removed the spent chemo bag and discarded it and all of the attached tubing into a medical waste disposal bin. Next, she brandished a syringe that looked to be the size of a small car. It was filled with a reddish-colored liquid and was labeled "idarubicin." I kid you not; it looked like the holding area in this syringe had a gallon of the reddish liquid ready for immediate dispatch. I hoped that they would offer some goofy juice before putting this stuff into me.

After some prep that included flushing my mediport with heparin, the business end of the huge syringe was attached to a tube hanging from my port. In a matter of thirty seconds or so I watched this liquid as it was forced by plunger out via the tubing and into my port. We had now deposited another chemical directly into my jugular. That was the first of the '3' in the '7+3' protocol of chemotherapy drugs I would receive.

My nurse seemed much too happy while doing that, and I wondered if she had a nighttime gig as an executioner. Not for money; just for fun.

Day one of chemotherapy was complete. That wasn't so bad, I thought, as I went for a walk accompanied by my trusty rolling IV stand. Hanging from the stand was a single clear bag of liquid something-or-other to keep me hydrated, and the IV pump that was not running for the time being. I vowed to walk every chance I got, as I felt that the fight had really just begun. I had every intention of walking away from the nightmare called AML just as soon as I was able; hopefully while the devil wasn't paying attention, just in case.

# Chapter 13

The same routine continued for two more days like clockwork. Vitals every four hours, port flush and blood draw for CBCs, and then breakfast consisting of coffee, juice and some fruit. Next was my walk for exercise, pre-chemo meds, the first chemo course of cytarabine, and then a syringe full of idarubicin to wash it down. I hardly touched lunch, as my appetite had gone somewhere on vacation. A walk, some television and a delivery from Rosemary the snack lady filled my afternoons. I picked at dinner but never really ate a whole meal. Terry spent her free time by my side and made a concerted effort to bring some regular food in from a local sandwich shop to try to stimulate my appetite.

So far, so good. Physically I felt fine, and I looked forward to the visits of a few close friends, along with phone calls and emails from my extended family. There were not a whole lot of other things to look forward to, other than getting cured and going back home to my life.

The next four days brought more of the same, minus the idarubicin booster. I still walked as far and as often as I could in order to keep the blood pumping. I met different nurses, CNAs, NSAs, doctors, clinicians, and housekeepers. I genuinely liked most everyone that I had the opportunity and privilege to meet. Each seemed proficient at their job, and more importantly, to love their work even in the face of the constant adversity that cancer delivers.

Dr. Rodriguez, or sometimes another oncologist from his practice, stopped by each day to observe the progress and results of my treatment. Hospitalists, staff doctors, or their representatives came by each day to observe and then record their own assessment of my present condition. Each had a unique approach and bedside manner. Some appeared really detached and aloof, and behaved as though I was just a nuisance blocking the progress of their daily routine. Others seemed empathetic and offered words of support and encouragement. Some offered explanations of the medical and lab tests I was being subjected to, and information about the medicines I was taking. All were willing to answer the many questions I had. I could only hope that I was asking the right ones.

I have to say, that after all I read and heard about chemotherapy, it had not seemed to affect me in any way, save for a lousy appetite. I actually wondered if I was some kind of special human who possessed a very inhuman tolerance to chemotherapy. I also hoped that the supposed healing power of these chemicals could somehow permeate my supernatural tolerance. I began this treatment as folically challenged so I didn't have much hair to begin with, but my mustache and eyebrows were hanging in there pretty much intact. I was led to believe that chemo would eradicate any remaining hair follicles. Perhaps alopecia will also be defeated by my new superpowers. I was actually feeling pretty cocky about all this.

I had gotten to know my nurses and aides on a very personal level, or perhaps I should say they knew too much about me and I, in return, tried to learn more than just their names. I tried to learn something personal about each of my caregivers, and what I learned sometimes gave great insight into why they were such caring and wonderful individuals, and why they chose this calling.

When Katie, the floor supervisor, hinted to Terry and me that more chemo was about a month away, we looked at each other with a knowing glance. We wondered how naive Katie was for a person in charge of all that happens here, on this battlefield so close to heaven, but even closer to hell. We forgave her; she is young. Dr. Rodriguez said four weeks and out. Period. End of story. The four-week odyssey alone will dictate life or death from leukemia. Either the chemo does its magic and life goes on, or it doesn't. No do-over, no what did Katie call it, consolidation therapy? Bone marrow transplant was a subject that was only brought up if everything else failed. Or so I thought.

Other nurses hinted at consolidation therapy as well, and not just one session, but possibly as many as three. Three more? You've got to be kidding. I needed to see Dr. Rodriguez, right away! I was finally beginning to see a pattern develop. Oh, how dumb could I possibly have been? After countless hours of research and study I somehow missed the part about consolidation chemotherapy. I'm certainly not a genius, but I do consider myself to be of reasonable intelligence, and I wonder how this could have been overlooked or ignored. No matter, things are going so well that I guess we would deal with consolidation therapy at a later date.

# Chapter 14

*Trouble is brewing*

Around 3:00 p.m. my vitals were taken. The CNA said that I was running a temperature of 100.5°. This wasn't terrible news, but if it got any higher, they would have to investigate the cause. A doctor decided that I must have a chest X-ray right away. They will use the chest X-ray taken prior to mediport implant surgery on April 19th as a comparator. Results offer no clues.

Over the next 24 hours, my fever escalated to a temperature of 102.9°. This was despite the IV additions of vancomycin and cefepime. Both are antibiotics used to treat serious bacterial infections. I also received the attention of a new doctor; he is from the Infectious Disease Control (IDC) department and was apparently an addition to my fast-growing payroll. Blood cultures were drawn in an attempt to discover the cause of the fever.

Lab test results showed my white blood count (WBC) at 0.3 (normal is 4.2 - 10.0), and platelets at 27,000 (normal is 140,000 - 440,000). Blood cultures exhibited no growth so far. An additional chest X-ray indicated no active disease. I was screwed for sure.

The next few days proved that the only person making a correct assumption was me; I was 100% correct when I said, "I was screwed for sure." We went from just a fever, to a fever plus something called "red man syndrome." Nobody was calling it that, but I later discovered that someone probably should have. My legs and arms began to swell until they resembled sausages. Within a day or so, my skin developed a red rash. The swelling then spread like a helium tank was attached to my mediport, and the red rash began to claim all available real estate. All of my caregivers began to look very concerned. No humor was offered, and that scared me. I could always count on somebody to make a joke about something and I could laugh right along with them. Often I instigated the humor, but suddenly I wasn't feeling much like a comedian.

Let's review. A few days ago, I completed a 7+3 chemo protocol with no obvious side effects, except perhaps some boredom with my daily routine. Now I lay here in bed, my skin a bright red, splotchy tarp pulled tightly in all directions like the cover of a snare drum. Add to this the additional grotesque swelling of my mouth, nose and eyes and you begin to see the picture. Adding even more to my misery, new doctors appeared randomly to take a quick look and to check vitals. Maybe there is a cash pool in the doctor's lounge and they need to get a first-hand look in order to place an informed bet. I'd like to get a piece of the action and bet that I'll see a bright light within 24 hours. This really sucked. The worst part was the look on Terry's face; a look that I will never forget. I have never seen her look quite so worried.

Terry told the nurses and all of the doctors that the first signs of rash and swelling were within the first few hours after beginning infusion of the antibiotic cefepime. Terry is smart like this and possesses an unusually strong and accurate common sense. She sees what many of us miss and instinctively knows what to do about it. She wants the cefepime removed from my medications, yet nobody will take her seriously. How could she possibly know more than all of these doctors?

I read many months later that red man syndrome[3] is considered a common reaction to

---

[3] Ref: http://www.ncbi.nlm.nih.gov/pmc/articles/PMC270616/

vancomycin but not to cefepime. Red man syndrome is a hypersensitivity reaction often associated with rapid infusion of the first dose of the drug, and was initially attributed to impurities found in vancomycin preparations. Other antibiotics or drugs that stimulate histamine release can also result in red man syndrome.

We may never know for certain whether the source of my red man syndrome was vancomycin, cefepime, or something unrelated to either of those antibiotics.

# Chapter 15

The following few pages identify actions taken on my behalf and the care, radiology and imaging performed. The dates, times and comments are real, not imagined. The large package containing my medical records from 2011 was used as reference to make sure that I did not exaggerate or mistakenly remember something different from actual events and reality. Terry tells me that 'chemo-brain' is a residual effect from my treatments and that I should be vigilant to ensure that any imagined fantasy does not creep onto my stage of reality.

May 2, 2011 11:42 a.m.

Off to radiology for a 'CT-guided bone marrow biopsy'. This procedure was painless and did not compare to the biopsy performed on the run in Dr. Rodriguez's office a few weeks ago. What a difference a few million dollars invested in capital equipment can make. This biopsy will indicate the current status of my leukemia, and if the chemotherapy has accomplished the intended results.

May 2, 2011 7:37 p.m.

My swelling was the same, the rash was worse and the medications continued unchanged. Off to radiology again. This time it was for a chest X-ray. Apparently everything was normal, and the report I read later said there was no acute cardiopulmonary disease, but there were degenerative changes in the spine. Why didn't anybody tell me what they were really looking for? Instead of helpful information, I was offered platitudes similar to "We just want to see what's going on." I decided to trust nobody at this point except Dr. Rodriguez and my nurses.

May 3, 2011 Morning

Good news / Bad news. The good news: I was in remission! The bone marrow biopsy showed that I had no remaining sign of leukemia. The bad news: leukemia patients usually die of a peripheral or residual disease or cancer caused, at least in part, by the damage that chemotherapy heaped upon your major organs.

I was struggling with red man syndrome and fevers, and I wondered to which I would succumb. Would I continue to swell until my skin exploded and they found my blood and guts stuck to the wallpaper, floor and ceiling? Or would the infection that was causing my fever just take over and kill me slowly?

I chose neither. I would fight this to the best of my ability. I would like to see my grandson again. The framed pictures put together by Stacy and John that sat on top of the chest of drawers beside my bed were a constant reminder of what lied beyond this treatment. I vowed to beat this, so bring it on.

May 3, 2011 2:13 p.m.

Off to radiology again. A 'CT chest w/o contrast' was ordered.

May 4, 2011

I received a consultation from yet another new doctor. "Impression is acute kidney injury, nonoliguric," whatever that meant. I'll look it up later. The report also noted nephrotoxicity from antibiotics, specifically vancomycin and amphotericin. I'm trying to stay away from the medical terminology; please bear with me and I promise there will be no surprise quiz.

Vancomycin and amphotericin were both discontinued; the rash and swelling had not abated. I was not even aware that I was being treated with amphotericin. Terry told me later that I was not cognizant of my circumstance or surroundings for much of this week.

May 4, 2011 4:13 p.m.

Off for an ultrasound. 'Renal sonogram to investigate suspected kidney injury' as ordered.

May 5, 2011

I couldn't seem to shake the hideous swelling and rash. Cefepime was still hanging on my IV stand because I needed antibiotics, and the vancomycin and amphotericin that were found to possibly have created nephrotoxicity were removed. I was on my way to the OR for an excisional biopsy to be taken from my lower back. This meant that nobody could yet answer the burning question "Why does Johnny have swelling and a rash?" So, let's cut out some skin.

A 5.2cm layer of skin was removed for pathology and cultures. The only good part about that procedure, from my point of view, was the goofy juice. Have I mentioned before that I like goofy juice? The area from where the biopsy was taken was stitched up and covered with a two-by-three inch gauze pad.

That area on my back would bleed under a bandage and gauze for months to come. Every time the bandage was removed for replacement, skin would tear off with it and cause fresh bleeding. It could not heal properly because I had such a low platelet count.

May 5, 2011 7:00 p.m.

Off to radiology for an 'MRI of the abdomen w/o contrast'. They needed to evaluate the left kidney. The ultrasound of May 4th was used as a comparison. I wondered what would possibly show up in the 26 hours since the comparison ultrasound.

I couldn't wait to get the bills for all of these procedures. If I were a car, I would have been thrown onto the scrap heap for sure, or maybe the lemon law would have spared us from further misery. I also wondered if the invoices for all of this care would be my legacy. I was having heart palpitations just thinking of the damn medical expenses piling up as fast as the national debt. Maybe I should have an EKG in addition to all of this!

May 6, 2011 5:06 p.m.

Off to radiology for my nightly soiree. This time it was for a 'Lung scan vent/perfusion' and the purpose was to rule out PE. Pulmonary Embolism[4] (PE) is a blockage of a major artery in the lung, while Pulmonary Edema (PE) is merely swelling; take your pick here, because I am not sure which we were looking for, but dollars to donuts it was the edema. Edema[4] results whenever small blood vessels become 'leaky' and release fluid into nearby tissues. The extra fluid accumulates, causing the tissue to swell. Sound familiar?

May 6, 2011 5:35 p.m.

I guess I needed another chest X-ray. They used the chest X-rays from May 2nd as a

---

[4] Definition from WebMD

comparison. Of course, they had many to choose from, but for the sake of continuity, they used that one. It appeared as though my heart was "mildly enlarged" according to the report I later read. Why didn't someone mention this, I wonder? The secrets were piling up, and I felt like an outsider with a limited-access pass.

May 7th must have been a holiday in radiology because I was not invited for my nightly scans. I did still have red man syndrome and nothing had changed. I still had a fever and the cefepime was still hanging on my IV stand, poisoning me slowly. By now, Terry had become a lot more vocal and assertive. She was insistent that the cefepime be removed. Nobody listened, nobody cared. I believe she had been right all along, but I equate this to "if a tree falls in the forest and no one is around to hear it, does it make a sound?"

May 8, 2011 9:53 a.m.

Off to radiology for yet another chest X-ray. They were looking for infiltrates and acute cardiopulmonary disease, according to the report. The X-ray from May 6th was used as a comparison. They must have been looking for a very fast-moving something that wasn't there just a day and a half ago.

May 10, 2011 7:54 a.m.

Off to radiology. My check-in time at radiology was getting earlier each day. This worried me and I wondered why I got such priority booking times all of a sudden. This couldn't be good, although maybe I was starting to accumulate frequent flier points. Anyway, I had another 'chest X-ray (CHEST PA/LAT (CXR)'. The X-ray from May 8th was chosen for use as a comparison.

May 10, 2011 6:53 p.m.

Off to radiology once more. This time I had complained of stomach pain so we needed abdominal X-rays. I used to just take an antacid; my, how things have changed.

May 11, 2011 9:49 p.m.

Off to radiology for a 'CT sinuses w/o contrast' as we continued the quest to find a cause for my fever. This test ignored the continuing swelling and rash apparently. I resigned myself to the fact that I might resemble a strawberry for the balance of my time here on earth. I wondered if I should buy a battery for my watch or if it would be a waste of money. I wasn't sure at that point if I should even buy green bananas.

A 'CT chest w/contrast' and a 'CT ABD/PEL W/&W/O CONTR 1+ REGNS' followed the CT sinus scan. The three additional CT scans were also on the lookout for something that may have been causing the fever.

I don't know what '1+REGNS' meant, unless it indicated 'more than one region'. We did have the chest, sinus, abdomen and pelvis represented here, as well as with *and* without contrast. That's a lot of bases to cover all at once, and I applauded the effort.

I wondered if they would name a hospital wing after me because of all the income I generated for the radiology department. My nurses said the only wing named for me would appear on a dinner plate accompanied by dipping sauce.

# Chapter 16

*Friday the 13th*

Friday, May 13, 2011

Sometime within the last 24 hours, cefepime had been removed from my intravenous diet. I hadn't noticed it missing from my IV tower. I wondered if the appearance of a new doctor from IDC had something to do with the cefepime removal, or if Terry had taken it down on her own. My medical records don't mention who ordered the deletion of this antibiotic.

Regardless of who was responsible, or why the cefepime had been discontinued, my swelling and rash were beginning to subside. I was thankful, and Terry finally felt some sense of vindication. If the original IDC doctor had discontinued the cefepime, maybe we could have avoided a large chunk of the imaging and radiology testing costs incurred since May 2<sup>nd</sup>. Maybe the excisional biopsy taken from my back would have been avoided as well.

The bottom line was that I was feeling much better and couldn't wait to get home and leave that nightmare in my rear view mirror. So much for trixadexaphobia. I now consider Friday the 13<sup>th</sup> as my lucky day.

# Chapter 17

May 14, 2011

The world seemed a better place today. The swelling and rash all but disappeared overnight. I saw a light at the end of this tunnel, and just hoped it was not attached to a freight train. I sensed relief on the faces around me, and Terry was smiling for the first time in a week or two. The usual parade of doctors continued, but even they seemed relieved. Dr. Rodriguez just shook his head and said, "Welcome back."

For the first time since I can't remember when, I was hungry. Terry brought in a hot meatball sub and potato chips from the sandwich shop downstairs. We shared the meal mostly in silence, both of us wondering what was around the next corner.

My fever subsided for the better part of the day, but the 4:00 p.m. vitals check told us that the fever is not done with me just yet. The doctors were hinting that I could go home if I could avoid a fever for 24 hours. It was good to have a goal, and I hoped that the fever would stay away for just one day. One step at a time; I'll cross the next bridge when I get there.

May 15, 2011

Overnight vitals revealed no fever and I was excited because I was looking at discharge before the day was out. The IDC doctors were suddenly not sure they agreed that I should go home, however, and we had a lengthy discussion about their opinion. The small army of my other doctors had agreed that I was good to go, but the final decision belonged to IDC. I needed to get out of there; I knew I'd be OK, if only I could get back to my life at home. Finally, the IDC doctors agreed to this, as long as my 4:00 afternoon vitals were within acceptable limits and I had a normal body temperature.

Against all the rules, Terry agreed to bring in some Tylenol for me that afternoon. The plan was to take a few of those to disguise any sign of fever. No fever, and I'd be sprung for sure. I realized that was very wrong, but felt if I didn't get out of there soon, I may never leave at all.

The Tylenol was in my system a good 30 minutes before the CNA appeared with her work cart. Blood pressure, oxygen and heart rate were at acceptable levels, and I held my breath as my temperature registered on the ear probe thermometer with an audible beep that would determine my future. We were surprised and delighted that my body temperature was normal. This was in the bag now; we're out of here!

"Not so fast," was the response from the IDC doctors. Crap. They were trying to renege on our deal and I was not a happy camper. They said there had not been enough time without fever to allow me to get my life back. I find it ironic that the same people who, in my mind, caused a lot of my issues because of their inability to listen should have the final say here. We had a deal and now they're trying to back out. That was unacceptable; I was angry and I let them know. A long conversation ensued, and our negotiating resulted in a promise of discharge in the morning. That was the best that I could do, and if my fever returned the deal was off.

I'll tell you this; my fever would not return. The Tylenol in my drawer would see to that. Although I fully realized that disguising an underlying fever while neutropenic was not intelligent, I didn't care. I knew that if I could just go home that I would be OK. I couldn't spend another day in this place.

May 16, 2011

Vitals in the morning were within normal limits, including body temperature. IDC agreed to discharge me, but with a prescription for an antibiotic, Levaquin. I finished packing my belongings well before 5:00 a.m., showered, dressed and was ready to go. The sooner I got away from there, the better.

Terry showed up early, knowing I anticipated that moment for what seemed an eternity. My whole world was inside of that room for almost a month. The discharge paperwork was already prepared by my nurses; they also knew I needed to leave there as quickly as possible, and did their best to facilitate my departure.

We grabbed my belongings, discharge paperwork, the Levaquin script and we were off. Thank you, God. I insisted on walking out of there under my own power, and politely refused the offered wheelchair and escort. I was weak and a bit wobbly but Terry was there; we knew we could manage to do it together.

We stopped at a neighborhood pharmacy on the way home and Terry went in to pick up my prescription for Levaquin. Twenty minutes later, we had five (yes 5) pills for $175. Terry swore that they accepted the insurance card, but that was the price they charged her. I found the cost hard to believe, but I was too tired to care. We would deal with it later; I just wanted to go back to our home. The pharmacy was a preferred prescription provider for our insurance plan, but if we were overcharged I will 'unfriend' them in a heartbeat.

# Chapter 18

'Home, Sweet Home' is not just a sign hanging in the foyer anymore. It was great to be at home; I've not been that happy or so much at peace in some time. I felt weak as I walked up the stairs, but overwhelmed by a feeling of sweet relief that I made it that far. For a brief moment I wondered what the cost of the past four weeks would be, not to my health and well-being, but in dollars. I guess about $1 million should do it. How much will be covered by insurance is a question to be answered when the bills and Explanation of Benefits (EOBs) start to arrive. Judging by the cost of the five pill regimen of Levaquin we just paid, I'll be fortunate to keep the same home address. With the help of a glass of water, I ingested one of the five $35 pills and headed off to the bedroom to sleep. It is difficult to explain what a welcome sight my own bed was.

I reveled in my familiar surroundings, although I felt weak and noticed that much of my muscle mass had disappeared. My shoulders were droopy and my arms and legs looked like toothpicks with a thin layer of skin glued on. Terry can wrap my wrist in the grip of one of her hands and touch two fingers together. This was never even a remote possibility in the past. I've never been an exercise nut, but I tried to swim laps in a pool each day, and was accustomed to physical labor and sporting activities. Still, I was quite surprised at the horrible deterioration that had taken place. I promised myself that, as soon as I feel better and regain some strength, I'll work hard to get back into a reasonably fit physical condition.

The mediport implant was a visible lump beneath my skin and I had a band-aid over the area to help stop the bleeding caused when the needles were removed. The catheter beneath my skin running from the port to my jugular was clearly visible as well, especially where it was stitched in place just over the collarbone. My low platelet count was to blame for the bleeding. I needed be very careful with sharp objects, as a simple cut or tear in my skin could be the cause of continuous bleeding and would also create an opportunity for infection to step in.

I did not have a fever after my first night back at home. I don't know if it was due to the

Levaquin or was just a coincidence. My face felt 'funny', so I went to the bathroom vanity mirror. Staring back at me was a shadow of my former self, but with some massive swelling from cheekbone to lower jaw. I instinctively knew exactly what caused the swelling.

That was swelling I have experienced before. Not during my hospitalization, but long ago in my past. I had an abscessed tooth and was prescribed an antibiotic by my dentist. The swelling occurred when the abscess began to drain. A light bulb lit up brightly above my head, just like in the cartoons.

About three weeks before my first visit to Dr. Green with my complaint of dyspnea, I had a toothache resonating from an upper molar. There was minor swelling and a touch of pain, but they subsided in a day or two. I did not visit a dentist because I figured it might have been an irritation or small infection caused by a cut in the gum from a potato chip or other food. In any case, the tooth was no longer an issue and I quickly forgot about it. I'm now guessing that the handfuls of Motrin I was taking for my headaches may have temporarily relieved the pain and swelling.

The only parts of my body that did not receive one X-ray after another were my face and jaws. The sinus CT scan was the closest we got, but I wonder if anything would have shown up even if they were looking for it. Bottom line is that the tooth never hurt again, did not swell and I did not even think of it during my entire hospital stay. I am fairly certain that this tooth was the cause of what normally would have been just a low-grade fever had my immune system not been compromised. Case closed; seemingly endless radiology and testing procedures due to a minor tooth infection that started the snowball rolling downhill. Go figure.

Terry was horrified at the sight of the swelling and wanted to head directly back to the hospital. It took a while, but I was finally able to convince her that the sky was not falling. If, in a day or two, the swelling did not disappear, or if a fever started up, I would go back to the hospital to have it checked out. For now, I wanted to remain in my home and let this thing run its course. Like I said, I had seen this before. It's not that I'm smart; it's just the product of wisdom that has grown from the seeds of my previous experience.

Sure enough, over the course of the next two days, the swelling seemed to slide down away from the cheekbone and disappear into my lower jaw until there was no hint that it was ever present. I needed to remember that Levaquin did this trick for me, and I filed it in my memory banks right alongside goofy juice.

# Chapter 19

My hair was falling out at an alarming rate, not that there was much to begin with. Actually, I learned that my hair follicles became extremely brittle, so brittle that the individual hairs were breaking off, not falling out. In a week my body would be host to less hair than a cue ball. I was OK with that; it was a small price to pay and I wasn't vain to begin with. I do understand how women would feel given the same issue however, and I empathized with them.

Thursday, May 26th, I arrived at the hospital for a 9:00 a.m. CT-guided bone marrow biopsy. An NPO order began at midnight and stole away only my coffee because I don't usually eat breakfast on most days. There was a minimal wait, and the painless procedure was over within an hour.

One week later, I visited Dr. Rodriguez to have CBCs drawn and to receive an assessment of my condition. The marrow biopsy from the previous week was testament to my continuing remission. I am referred to as being CR-1; the 'CR' meaning 'complete remission.' Good news, for sure. The bad news is that Katie and the other nurses were absolutely correct when they subtly mentioned consolidation chemotherapy.

I did expect consolidation therapy after performing additional research when the subject first came up. I was surprised, however, when Dr. Rodriguez said the schedule was to go back to the hospital the very next Monday for a five day inpatient stay. I would receive a high-dose cytarabine chemo infusion on Monday, Wednesday and Friday. By high-dose, he meant a triple. Crap. What could go wrong this time?

On top of this, Dr. Rodriguez told me to expect the same each month for the next four months. Are you kidding? I could almost hear a flushing sound; there goes my business. I obtained substitute coverage for four or five weeks, and told each of my customers that I would return within five weeks to offer my personal service once again.

When I asked Dr. Rodriguez why I was not told about the whole plan, he pleaded *mea culpa* and said that most people can't handle the truth about all of this. He was trying to manage my feelings so as not to overwhelm me with the enormity of AML treatment. We agreed that full disclosure was required from here on, and I realized that my business may become a casualty of his well-meaning efforts to spare me the details.

To test Dr. Rodriguez's new policy of transparency and full disclosure, I began a brief Q&A dialogue:

Q. "I am in remission; what happens if I relapse?"

A. "We'll begin a new chemotherapy protocol."

Q. "What if I can't get to another remission?"

A. "You will die from leukemia."

Looks like Dr. Rodriguez was serious about this full disclosure stuff. I've created a monster.

# Chapter 20

The realization that my business was facing the firing squad proved to be correct. I contacted each customer individually to offer my apologies and to discuss the news of my new treatment plan. Many of my residential customers were more than understanding, and offered their encouragement and support. Some were angry, as they incorrectly believed I had intentionally misled them in order to avoid service cancellations. Most were willing to continue with my replacement, and I was grateful for their understanding. The commercial arm of the business was another matter.

My commercial business was just that; business. When it is business, feelings are irrelevant. There are schedules to be kept and work to be done. A few customers previously agreed to put their work on hold for four to five weeks, as long as I could pick up the slack upon my return. With the news of my new treatment plans, they needed to assign the work to another vendor. My issues were mine alone, and not their problem. I let them down. I agreed; given the same circumstances I would bid this vendor goodbye despite any personal feelings. Business is business, as we all know.

One commercial customer, a bank that I held in especially high esteem, wished me well and offered their business to me again in the future should I ever become well enough to continue. Though I appreciated the offer, I think we both knew that my return would not be possible unless my replacement performed in a grossly incompetent manner. To vet and hire someone for that work was an expensive proposition, and although I'm a nice guy and did a great job for them, once I was replaced the script was written. The time and effort expended during the past three years to build a business and the trust required to retain it just vanished in front of my eyes.

When I met with the interim replacement for my residential business, it became clear that continuing service for my customers was not going to work for him. He had a business of his own and needed to cater to his own customers; not to mine. I begged, pleaded and was finally able to cajole him into taking on my customers as his own, and to use my pricing schedules that were somewhat different than his. I did not attempt to sell my customers or my business; I only wanted to honor the trust that my customers gave to me when we agreed upon schedules and pricing. Many of my residential agreements were sealed with only a handshake. I always considered those handshakes to be a moral and ethical obligation, and it was important to me that my word to take care of them be honored, leukemia or not. I breathed a huge sigh of relief when an agreement was reached. Unfortunately, I would never see any benefit or reward for my work from building that business, or for the trust I upheld for the past several years.

# Chapter 21

The following day, I accepted delivery of a hypodermic needle containing an injection of Neulasta. Neulasta is a variant of the generic pegfilgrastim, a white cell booster. It is used to stimulate the growth of healthy white blood cells in the bone marrow after chemotherapy treatment. I needed to self-administer the 6mg injection 24 hours after the upcoming week of consolidation chemotherapy ended. The syringe required refrigeration until thirty minutes prior to injection before being allowed to warm to room temperature. The instruction sheet reminded me of the Sunday newspaper. How was anybody expected to read, comprehend and retain more than a page or two of this?

My eye was immediately drawn to bold print near the beginning of the document. Paraphrased, the injection contained a biotechnology-produced protein that used E. coli. Are you kidding? One common strain of E.

coli is O157:H7 that, in some people, may cause severe anemia or kidney failure, which can lead to death. I also found out E. coli already lives in your digestive tract.

What a great idea; deliver this potentially deadly bacterium in a very convenient hypodermic needle directly into the hands of someone who has never self-injected. What could possibly go wrong? I'm sure that I misunderstood the medical application of E. coli, and decided to investigate next week during my hospital stay.

My co-pay for the injection was $100, which seemed expensive. Boy, did I have a surprise in store! In the months to follow, I would break down EOB statements from the insurance company into manageable pieces. I saw the billed price, the insurance-negotiated discounts, my deductibles, co-pays and co-insurance dollar amounts. The *due from patient* line is my financial responsibility for the service or product listed and included the aforementioned deductibles, co-payments and co-insurance, plus any remaining uncategorized balance that has not been paid or otherwise offset with credits.

This 6mg injection had a *billed charge* of $9,031.05, and was discounted by 40% to an *allowed charge* of just $5,418.63, or about $903 per milligram.

During a search on the internet seeking information about Neulasta, I found that I received a bargain. Other cancer patients using that drug claim to have paid quite a bit more for an injection. In some cases I read, the cost was out of pocket and not covered by any insurance plan. Some of the examples were cited as originating in Canada, which I believe has national health care. Is this what I have to look forward to with Obamacare? Please say it isn't so, or just put me out of my misery now.

# Chapter 22

*Consolidation chemotherapy #1*

June 6, 2011

Monday morning, Terry unloaded me at the hospital inpatient registration department on her way to work. I had to wait an hour or so for the office to open, so I sat in the lobby and passed the time reading a paperback book I brought along for my five-day stay.

After registration and receiving my new patient bracelet, I made my way up to the oncology floor on 2-West. People think if you say *oncology* instead of *cancer* that it will be somehow less threatening. I knew my way around by now, so I politely declined the escort that was normally required for the elevator ride followed by a short walk past the surgical waiting room and orthopedics.

It felt like old home week when I entered the administration area of 2-West. There were lots of smiling faces and greetings from the nurses, CNAs, and secretarial and administrative friends I made during my last stay. I remain very fond of these people who spend their working days or nights here amid such misery and suffering. I'm not sure anyone working here realizes they each possess a heavenly gift. They willingly share this gift with so many patients that really, really need their care and understanding. I often think of them as the *Angels of 2-West*.

It's been three weeks since I left here but it seems like a lifetime. I still don't know, or perhaps I subconsciously refuse to acknowledge, the full extent of the horrors endured during my previous stay. I try not to dwell on it, though it is difficult to learn from something you are trying to forget.

Consolidation chemotherapy was considerably more convenient than my initial chemo treatments. Maybe it was my familiarity with the people and surroundings. Maybe it was because only chemo and a single bag of saline were hooked up to my mediport, and just for a few hours every other day. I must admit I did not miss the antibiotics and the radiology. I did hope the issue with my molar and the ensuing infection were history.

I was in good spirits for most of the week, and Terry was with me much of the time. I especially enjoyed the food she brought in from outside the cafeteria service system, and my appetite was healthy. I was now privy to the fact that some special off-menu items could be ordered from the NSAs for each meal. Pizza, cheeseburgers and taco salads had become my favorites. I guess I shouldn't call my appetite *healthy* when the staples of my diet were essentially junk food. There was a small kitchen that I raided for coffee, cups of chocolate or vanilla ice cream, orange sherbet, popsicles and snacks that were available any time, day or night. Cancer patients get all the good stuff.

Vitals at 4:00 a.m. and blood draws for CBCs at 5:00 had been combined into one visit around 5:00 a.m. This thoughtful rescheduling meant I now could sleep from midnight to 5:00 without interruption. Each day, I was wide awake shortly after sunrise, and took over the morning coffee-making duties from Cissy, the secretary. I didn't think she minded, and I really needed coffee when I awoke each day. I considered it cruel and unusual punishment to have to wait for my coffee.

By most accounts, I regarded the first consolidation week as a piece of cake compared to my initial chemo treatments. I was comfortable, in good spirits and maintained a very positive and optimistic outlook.

Terry dropped in every chance she got, and I knew how difficult these treatments were for her, although she never let on. Close friends continued to visit unannounced, but I informed others that a week-long therapy was in progress and a visit would be hit-or-miss as to my availability.

Though Terry and I are from very large extended families, we have no family here in Florida. Terry could use the support only family could offer at a time like this, but I didn't know if I could tolerate the look of pity in their eyes.

Terry is a very strong woman who does not like to share her emotions, and I suspected she would get through this in one piece. I do know the nurses kindly tried to boost her spirits. I also knew her crying and sadness would be confined to a dark room, alone in the still of night, in the shadows of what used to be our future together. My heart ached for her.

We were here in Florida because Mom & Dad were snowbirds from Massachusetts. They lived 8 or 10 miles from where Terry and I now call home, and owned a condo they occupied from October through April.

Dad passed away a few years back, so we came down here to live close enough to Mom to help out when needed, but not close enough to get under her skin. Mom enjoyed being on her own, and we were delighted to help out when needed. My sisters remained up north, other than taking short vacations here, and took care of her needs for the rest of the year.

Mom has since gone back up north to an assisted living facility. How ironic; we came to Florida to be near to her, now she has returned to New England and we are here alone. We bought our home during the real estate boom a few years back and are badly upside-down on our mortgage, so here we will remain for as long as the good Lord sees fit.

Discharge on Saturday, June 11th went off without a hitch. Vitals were taken and CBCs drawn at 5:00 a.m.; tubing and needles were removed from my mediport after the usual flush. My nurse and doctor friends completed all of the necessary paperwork. I was showered, dressed and out of there with Terry by 7:00. This discharge was fast and efficient, and I appreciated that everyone did their part to spring me from there early in the morning. I saw others wait for the better part of a day for their paperwork to be completed. It might have helped that I started reminding anybody who would listen on Wednesday that I was to be discharged on Saturday. It also might have helped that Terry and I always brought candy for the nurses; Reese's Peanut Butter Cups were their favorite, and we made sure there was always a supply on hand.

# Chapter 23

I was home, and it was about 24 hours after discharge from consolidation chemotherapy #1.

Reading about my self-injection of Neulasta was one thing, but when I was settled in around 11:30 a.m. on Sunday morning to actually perform the injection, I suddenly felt apprehensive. I read the instructions, but it did not occur to me to get personal instruction or practice when I was at the hospital. Now, I sure wish I had. I was ready to unload a small hypodermic injection with a discounted cost of more than $5400 that might just kill me if I screwed something up (remember the E. coli?).

Logic and calm prevailed; I administered the shot in my upper thigh exactly per the instructions. I had no problems; maybe there was a future for me in phlebotomy.

Monday morning I was at an appointment with Dr. Rodriguez for CBCs and a physical evaluation. My numbers looked OK, but I would still need to have CBCs drawn every other day. This requirement presented a small financial issue.

Whenever I visited with Dr. Rodriguez for an appointment, I would co-pay $60 as required by my insurance plan for a specialist visit. I was also expected, according to FCS, to provide the same co-pay when visiting this office, whether or not I was examined by Dr. Rodriguez. The same co-pay applied when I was there for a CBC blood draw done by their phlebotomists and the results evaluated by a nurse. This made no sense to me, and I argued my case to the business office. Although sympathetic, they offered only that I could call their main office for further clarification.

On the other hand, my insurance provided for CBCs at the hospital satellite blood draw locations at no charge. The only difference, $60 co-pay notwithstanding, was that results of CBCs drawn at the hospital blood draw centers are not available until that evening or the next morning. This was not acceptable, according to Dr. Rodriguez, because the test results might indicate a need for immediate treatment. $60 per visit ($180 each week) to have CBCs done at FCS is something I cannot afford to pay, as I was now out of work and had no income. We were at a stalemate, and I eventually decided that I would continue with CBCs drawn at a hospital draw center strictly because of the price tag.

On Wednesday I had CBCs drawn at a hospital draw center. If there were any issues raised because of the results, I didn't hear about them.

On Friday, I woke up with mouth sores that I've been told to expect because of low blood counts. Chemotherapy, through the lowering of blood counts, affects fast growing cells, and the mouth and throat are prime candidates, as are fingernails and hair. I had these white lesions, called thrush, on my tongue and on the inside surface of my cheeks. They were extremely uncomfortable and irritating, and I had great difficulty swallowing because of them. Eating food was out of the question.

Following instructions given me in the past by Dr. Rodriguez, I called his office to get a prescription for what is referred to as *magic mouthwash*. This was offered to me while in the hospital, but I had no need for it at the time. I called at 9:40 a.m. with this request and was told that somebody would call me back with the prescription information and details.

Shortly after 11:00 a.m. I was still waiting for my return phone call. Before I called back to remind them, I needed to use the bathroom. Imagine the shock when my urine appeared a bright, bright red! Nobody told me to expect this, and I was horrified. I immediately halted the flow of urine that I swore had to be pure blood. I knew I had not emptied my bladder, but was too afraid to continue. What would you do? I felt like I was urinating pure blood and wondered how much I could afford to pee away before I died due to a lack of the precious red fluid.

I immediately called Dr. Rodriguez's office to express my horror of what happened, and the fact that I now needed some quick help in addition to the magic mouthwash. "Don't worry, we'll get you some help," said the voice on the other end of the phone line. I was told to stay near the phone because somebody would call me right back. Reluctantly, I hung up the telephone, though I felt like I was rolling the dice on a craps table that might never pay out.

Soon enough though, I received a phone call from someone at the office instructing me to go to the transfusion center the next day to receive a platelet transfusion. A low platelet count had apparently allowed blood to enter my bladder. This was getting to be a thrill a minute and I silently wondered, once again, what will be next?

The next day I kept my appointment at the LMHS transfusion center as arranged by FCS and received a unit of platelets. I had thrush in my mouth that still needed to be addressed, but in comparison to bright red urine, it wasn't that big of a deal.

# Chapter 24

To this day, I fail to understand the business relationship between Lee Memorial Health System and Florida Cancer Specialists, if indeed one exists. It's not that I *need* to understand, but I really would *like* to understand because knowing might help with my decision making as I try to navigate through the maze of red tape I keep running into.

The Regional Cancer Center building in the geographic area referred to as the 'Sanctuary' has smaller lettering under the main title that reads 'Lee Memorial Health System'. On the first floor there is a reception area, some doctor's offices, radiology and radiation suites, and a small deli. On the second floor is the LMHS transfusion center, phlebotomy lab, cancer nurse offices and administrative personnel. I'm sure there are many more offices and meeting rooms, but I am not aware of what those other rooms might contain. The third floor houses the offices of Florida Cancer Specialists, and also a transfusion center, as well as doctor offices and a phlebotomy lab. I've never been to the fourth floor, I don't know what is up there, and to be honest, I'd like to keep it that way.

The second floor is apparently owned, operated and staffed by the Lee Memorial Health System. My insurance plan requires that any transfusions be done there, on the second floor. Fair enough; I understand the need for cost control. They are also equipped to perform CBC blood draws with stat results, that is to say, results are immediately available. But not for me; I must go elsewhere for blood draws.

Florida Cancer Specialists occupies the third floor, and has a transfusion center that I am not allowed to use, also by virtue of insurance rules. Additionally, if I have CBCs drawn at FCS on the third floor I am required to front the $60 co-pay.

So exists this conundrum. I am not allowed to have a CBC blood draw at LMHS on the second floor that will offer the stat turnaround that Dr. Rodriguez requires. I must travel ¼ mile down the street to an outpatient draw center also owned and staffed by LMHS, but that does not offer a stat turnaround of results. This is because the blood samples are sent elsewhere for testing. I cannot use the FCS transfusion center on the third floor, and must use the second floor LMHS transfusion center to receive blood products. It sure seems to me that a little bit of teamwork may be necessary here. How difficult could it be to fix this?

Monday, June 20th, I went to the third floor to see Dr. Rodriguez and have CBCs drawn at the same time ($60 co-pay, but a visit with Dr. Rodriguez). Two hours later I was on the second floor for a platelet transfusion; $0 co-pay, but no CBCs. Dr. Rodriguez remained insistent that the CBC results be available immediately in case a transfusion was necessary, but at that time, the only place that could offer the required immediacy was FCS on the third floor.

I became quite vocal during my visits to the second floor facility about my inability to get CBC blood draws with stat results, rather than having to travel to another facility to get overnight-only results or paying $60 on the third floor. A sympathetic nurse volunteered to get involved. Her name was Malise and I made a mental note to send her supervisor or director a letter that would complement her willingness to become involved on my behalf. This is rare indeed, and I certainly appreciated all of her efforts, regardless of the outcome.

# Chapter 25

Tuesday, June 21, 2011

I reported to the Regional Cancer Center second floor transfusion center, this time for a transfusion of two units of blood. I was again reminded of the generosity of blood donors and silently gave thanks to each of them. In at 10:30 a.m. and out at 4:00 meant that I enjoyed yet another 'free' lunch.

Wednesday, I returned to receive a unit of platelets. This had become a habit and I wondered what the future might hold. It can't be good to receive blood and platelets almost every day. When will my immune system recover and start to make its own blood and platelets? Would I become forever dependent on donated blood products? What if I developed a resistance to donor blood products and my immune system started to reject them? What if there was a shortage of donated blood? Who is first in line? I think children who need blood products should get them first in the event there are not enough to go around. I would gladly forego donated blood products for myself if it gave a chance of life to a child who might otherwise not survive.

Friday brought with it an 8:00 a.m. appointment to get two units of blood followed by a 1:15 appointment up on the third floor with Dr. Rodriguez for CBCs and a physical evaluation.

Monday, June 27th

CBCs at FCS at 8:00 a.m.; additional $60 co-pay but Dr. Rodriguez needed results immediately. There did appear to be some movement in the efforts to have CBCs drawn at the second floor transfusion center instead of FCS or a LMHS blood draw station. Nurse Malise of the transfusion center had somehow arranged for this to happen; all we needed now was a doctor's order for this to become the real deal. A few minutes with Dr. Rodriguez's staff and this should be a reality.

FCS faxed orders to the transfusion center as requested. My Wednesday and future CBCs will now be drawn at the transfusion center; theoretically at least.

Wednesday, June 29th

I arrived at the second floor transfusion center for the CBC blood draw, but was informed that Dr. Rodriguez's orders were not specific enough. Apparently they did not specify the word '*stat*' and therefore I was out of luck. Everybody knew I needed a blood draw, everyone realized the results were needed right away, yet nobody could make that happen. I was really tired of fighting the red tape, so I surrendered and walked up to the third floor to fork over the $60 co-pay to have my CBCs drawn. After a short wait in the rear waiting room, a nurse appeared and told me I may go home; all was fine with my blood work.

Friday, July 1st

Today was CBCs and a visit with Dr. Rodriguez at FCS. The good news was that my blood counts recovered and were holding in the OK range. I did not need a transfusion of blood products for the time being. The bad news was that we're going to do this consolidation thing all over again. Rinse and repeat. Consolidation chemotherapy #2 would be another five days as an inpatient beginning on Monday, July 11th.

Friday, July 8, 2011

Today I received a home delivery of the Neulasta shot I needed to self-administer after discharge following my new week of consolidation therapy. The delivery was scheduled for yesterday, because I normally allowed extra time in case of unforeseen problems or delays. When I called Thursday at 4:45 p.m. to inquire about the delivery that had not yet arrived, I was informed that "they'll be there." When I inquired as to how late they might deliver, I received a curt, "They will be there when they get there; they are not finished for the day until they are done with deliveries." Duh. She did not even ask for my name.

You guessed it; there was no delivery as scheduled. When I complained the next morning, nobody knew about or could even find my order, nobody remembered talking to me, and certainly the person I spoke with would not take responsibility, and even denied speaking with me. Par for the course. They pretended the rude person in Customer Service was a figment of my imagination.

After lengthy discussion with a manager, it was arranged that an 'emergency' delivery would be made today. "Gee, we're sorry." Funny, I thought, you sounded the same when you were happy.

# Chapter 26

*Consolidation chemotherapy #2*

Monday, July 11, 2011

I presented myself to the registration desk at 8:00 a.m. with my duffle bag full of books, pajamas, laptop computer and treats (read: bribes) for the nursing staff and aides as usual. The drill hadn't changed and I waded quickly through the necessary paperwork and made my way directly up to the cancer floor on 2-West.

I was greeted warmly upon arrival by the unit secretary, nurses, and other staff members who happened to be at or near the reception area. Everything seemed so familiar, everybody was wearing a genuine smile, and I felt as though I was checking in at a nice hotel. I again thought to myself that these people really *are* angels sent here to protect me from the reality of cancer, and my mood was good. With these people on my side, how can I not beat this cancer?

My new home was a corner room overlooking the medical helicopter landing zone. I knew from past experience that the helipad is a busy piece of real estate, and I looked forward to the diversion that helicopter take-offs and landings would offer. I quickly unpacked and stored my clothing in the closet and chest of drawers, then arranged my toiletries on a metal shelf under the bathroom mirror. I liked the private room (all of the rooms are private on this floor) and still appreciated having a private bathroom and shower.

My day shift nurse stopped in within the first few minutes of my arrival. We exchanged pleasantries and caught up with what was new for both of us. I offered treats of peanut butter cups and some baked goods that Terry had packed for me. Terry thinks of everything.

During my first consolidation chemotherapy last month, one of my nurses prepared duplicate folders of completed paperwork that I would need to present each time I arrived as an inpatient. Included were the standard in-processing forms, medical and legal disclosures, personal property declarations, privacy notices, a living will and my health care proxy. The first time we sat to fill out and collect all of these forms and the signatures required to make them legal, it must have taken a half-hour or more. Thanks to the foresight and efficiency of that nurse, the whole ordeal was complete in seconds, as I needed only to present one of the duplicate set of documents so thoughtfully provided.

In short order, my vital signs of heart rate, blood pressure and body temperature were measured and recorded. My mediport was accessed, and two nurses were singing their duet as they verified the information on my wristband and double-checked that the cytarabine I was about to receive was the correct prescription and volume. I was pre-medicated with Decadron and Zofran orally to deal with the expected nausea and other side effects. I received steroid eye drops in an application that was repeated every six hours, gave a signature sample for later comparison, and got a hook-up to some IV fluids. It's as though we performed this routine one hundred times before. In reality, it had been a few dozen instances, including my initial stay and first consolidation therapy.

Five or ten minutes after the IV pump was programmed and started there was a problem, as indicated by the pump alarm. This *beep-beeping* was as annoying as I remembered it to be. Response time from the nurses to address the alarm was slow, and I had learned to silence the alarm by pressing an 'alarm acknowledge' button on the membrane keyboard. I figured that I wasn't going anywhere soon, so why put up with the racket? I'd just hit the nurse call-button at my bedside and let the voice on the other end know that there was a problem, and would you please send someone to address the issue?

That arrangement worked well for a while, but we experienced a lot of problems with that pump. It soon became irritating to me and to the nurses who had other patients to attend to. The last nurse to answer a call for help fixed the problem that was causing the alarm by changing out some tubing and connectors for a new set. She also explained to me that I should not silence the alarm; someone will hear it and deal with it as soon as they are able. "Fine," I offered, "but I'm the one who is a foot away from this thing as it *beep-beeps* for a half-hour before the issue can be addressed." For some reason, the nurse could not see the logic in my plea/statement and chose to alter the IV pump software characteristics so that the alarm could not be silenced by pressing a key. I now saw this as a challenge.

Sure enough, I easily found a rocker switch on the rear panel of the pump near the electrical power connection. It was labeled with a very small print that read "alarm reset." I really could have used more of a challenge here. In any case, a nurse appeared just as the last of the chemo from the plastic container was emptied into my port, and before the alarm would signal the session completion. I would have to put my research off until Wednesday, my next scheduled day for infusion.

I didn't feel any different after this infusion of chemo than I felt at any time during the previous few weeks. Good sign or bad, I am not sure. The afternoon and evening passed quietly and uneventfully, and I made sure to walk the hallways to get at least some sort of exercise.

I got into a routine and used a repetitive walking route, and followed it religiously. First, it was down to the 'U'-shaped dead end of the corridor where a locked door prevented entry to the roof. It was labeled "authorized personnel only," so I would turn around and continue on my route. Next, it was back the entire hallway length towards the 2-West entry area and through the hallways of orthopedics. Everyone up and about in orthopedics had a tubular aluminum walker or crutches or a wheelchair to aid in their mobility. Next, I would walk past the large surgical waiting room filled with anxious family members and friends, then up and right back down a few flights of stairs that nobody seemed to use. When I was attached by tubing to a rolling IV stand I could not use the stairs, but otherwise my route remained pretty much the same. I guess it was a feeble grasp for some form of continuity or routine. Maybe I could trick myself into believing that I actually had some say in the otherwise strict, no-compromise environment.

As I neared the end of my walk that day and heard all of the IV pump alarms loudly competing for attention, an idea came to mind. I had better write the idea down on paper, I thought, before it died of loneliness.

# Chapter 27

*Funny business*

Tuesday morning I had nothing going on, and after making coffee in the small kitchen and completing my walk for exercise, I returned to my room. I learned the IV pump alarm would activate any time a program was started and there was no flow of liquid through the small pump. After turning the machine on and starting a program to run, indeed the alarm began to sound off, so I quietly closed the heavy door to my room and began my sinister plan.

First, I opened an app on my smartphone that records voice and sound. While the pump alarm was wailing *beep-beeep, beep-beeep*, I initiated the sound recording and continued to record for about one minute. I saved the file, and then turned off the alarm and pump. Before shutting the pump down, I verified that the small rocker switch spotted earlier would indeed silence the alarm as I believed, at least for five minutes or so.

The balance of Tuesday disappeared in a blur of daytime television, responding to emails and reading part of a novel.

Wednesday morning, blood was drawn for CBCs at the end of the night shift. After my morning walk, I took the time to make some strong coffee using the stainless steel coffee maker in the kitchenette. The coffee tasted really bad, but I enjoyed the kick caffeine delivered. I also made a pot of decaffeinated coffee for others who might prefer less of a jolt from their hot morning beverage.

Following a breakfast of fruit and juice served bedside, two day shift nurses arrived to prep me for my chemo session. The handwriting sample, steroid eye drops and Tylenol, Decadron and Zofran pills were dispensed quickly. The nurses sang the chemo duet to verify the particulars of my high-dose cytarabine and my identity, in case some bad guy switched medical bracelets during the night shift in order to steal my chemo away. I still chuckled every time I saw the skull and crossbones symbol on an orange background labeling my medicine container.

Next, a length of clear tubing was connected to the IV pump and to my port, and then a saline IV was connected directly from the bag to a second mediport connection. The pump program was checked, and the pump was started.

I was prepared to have some fun with my nurses. I had my cell phone ready beneath the bed sheets; the pump alarm recording was queued up and ready to play on command.

As soon as the nurses turned away and headed for the door, I activated the alarm recording; *beep-beeep, beep-beeep*, loud and clear. The nurse nearest to the pump, Dee Dee, turned around to see what the problem was. I silenced the recording just as she reached for the pump shut-off switch and she stopped dead in her tracks.

"Gee," she said, "that's odd," and walked away. I immediately started to play the alarm recording again and Dee Dee stopped, turned to me and asked rhetorically, "I wonder what's up with this machine today?" as she reached for the off-switch. And, of course, I was just fast enough to silence the recording before her finger could hit the switch.

Dee Dee was perplexed, and I was grinning ear to ear; this was fun! The other nurse, Jonelle, witnessed this twice now from the doorway and was amused as well. She noticed the grin on my face and I thought she knew something was up. I signaled to her with the international 'shhh' gesture by holding a finger up to my pursed lips. Jonelle nodded, and instantly became my willing accomplice.

Dee Dee carefully inspected all of the pump and medicine bag connections as Jonelle and I watched, and then she checked to make sure that an air bubble was not present somewhere in the tubing. Once more, she walked towards the door; this time with an ear tuned in and waiting for the alarm to sound. Dee Dee appeared mystified and perhaps a bit shaken as she mumbled something under her breath.

You may have guessed by now that I quickly activated the recording again, *beep-beeep, beep-beeep*. This noise was annoying to begin with, but poor Dee Dee really had enough of that sound now. She performed an abrupt about-face, and then stormed towards the pump with her fists clenched and a look on her face that I'll never forget.

You must understand that Dee Dee is one of the kindest, most gentle people I ever met, but at this moment in time she looked like a pressure cooker ready to explode. Her face was beet-red with tiny droplets of sweat beginning to appear on her skin, and her breathing had become a bit irregular. She was obviously about to lose control.

Looking on, Jonelle, now joined by nurse Renee who heard the commotion from the hallway, couldn't hold it in any longer and began to laugh out loud. Dee Dee turned and seemed ready to smack Jonelle for laughing at her misfortune, but stopped when Renee and I began to laugh as well. It was now apparent that this had been a joke at Dee Dee's expense, and she laughed as well. It was a joy to see these three angels laughing; when I think of all the misery they witness every day, it is more than a small miracle they are even capable of laughter at all.

# Chapter 28

The rest of consolidation chemotherapy #2 went by quickly. Again, pestering everybody to make sure that my discharge paperwork was prepared well in advance has paid dividends. Thank you all; I'm out of here, see you next month for consolidation #3.

By the time Saturday afternoon rolled around, 24 hours had passed since my chemo infusions for consolidation #2 were complete. It was time again for my Neulasta shot to be self-administered. I really hated doing this, and I was nervous each time. I wonder how much damage could actually be caused if I screwed this up? Regardless of my feelings, my white cells need the boost Neulasta provides, so I stuck the needle into my thigh and just got it over with. When the hypodermic needle reservoir was empty, I placed the used hardware in a medical waste container provided and included in the delivered price of the drug.

Monday morning I was at FCS for CBCs. My numbers were low, but not low enough to need a blood or platelet transfusion. Rinse and repeat with identical results for Wednesday, but Friday I needed platelets. Arrangements were made for me to receive the platelets on the second floor transfusion center later in the day. It would take a few hours to obtain a unit of platelets, have them irradiated and shipped to the transfusion center for my use.

The transfusion center on the second floor had not changed since my last visit. I still couldn't get stat CBCs because of the oodles of red tape, but they were adept and most efficient when it came to my blood and platelet transfusions. Today, however, was different, as I encountered some resistance at check-in. I was told by the familiar receptionist that I must go down to the main lobby to complete a new-patient registration packet, because I had never been here before.

The reality is that I received transfusions of blood and/or platelets in that facility seven times within the last 45 days. I discussed this dilemma with the receptionist and her co-worker. Although the co-worker seemed to remember my name, there was no computer record of my having visited the facility prior to that day. When I began to name each of the nurses from whom I had received transfusions and described the transfusion area in great detail, a cloud of uncertainty and a glimmer of recognition began to spread across each of their faces. When I showed them my smartphone calendar from last month that noted each of my appointments and visits, they actually began to believe me. "Unfortunately," they said, "procedure must be followed," so I must go down to the lobby to register as a new patient.

I was more than a little confused, and I asked if the migration of their record-keeping to an EMR (Electronic Medical Record) system might have something to do with the problem. They seemed surprised that I was aware of this transition, and offered that perhaps it may have affected my medical records here. Regardless, I was told, I should go downstairs and re-register. Talk about red tape. . .

Down one flight of stairs (as I still tried to avoid the elevator) to the lobby, and I found the reception area barren of personnel. I did see someone in a connected area talking on the telephone, so I waited patiently for her to complete her call.

After what only seemed an eternity, she came forward to the reception desk and asked what I needed. When I said that I had to register as a new patient for the second floor transfusion center, she asked why I would need to register, as she recognized me from previous visits. She surrendered when I attempted to explain, and handed me a thick new-patient packet. I was directed towards an area with tables and chairs so I could sit down and attend to the paperwork details.

When I brought the completed package back to the reception desk, some carbon copies were extracted, and I was instructed to return the remains to the second floor receptionist.

Returning upstairs to the transfusion center reception area, I found the original receptionist missing, having been replaced by another. She greeted me with a friendly "Hi John, welcome back, do you have an appointment today?" I could only laugh or cry at that point. I settled for the former so she wouldn't make fun of me in the break room later in the day.

A few hours and one unit of platelets later, I was on my way home. I wondered out loud in the privacy of my car whether or not I should dispute the thousands of dollars in charges accrued previously, since I was a new patient? "Good luck with that," I told myself.

# Chapter 29

*Some days you're the windshield;*
*Some days you're the bug*

Allow me to introduce nadir. Nadir is a doozy, and is always to be expected after a chemotherapy session. When your blood counts are at their lowest, you are considered to be 'in your nadir'. This is the time when the marrow isn't making as many neutrophils, so your blood has far fewer of them traveling through your body. You are *neutropenic*. You may also be *anemic* due to a lack of red blood cells. To top it off, you may also have a condition called *thrombocytopenia* that occurs when you don't have enough platelets.

For me, nadir always occurred eight to ten days after my last infusion of chemo. It was then I felt the worst, and when I needed help by receiving transfusions of blood and/or platelets and/or Neupogen or Neulasta injections to stimulate white cell production.

Chemotherapy, as I understand it, is cumulative; sort of. It has been described to me by Dr. Rodriguez as a 'down' stairway where, each time chemo is infused, the body does not tolerate it as well as the previous instance. This stairway is one that you may only go down, so I guess that the *effects* of chemo are cumulative but the chemo itself eventually dissipates as it passes through your system.

Let's fast-forward to Monday, July 25th. I had an 8:30 appointment at FCS for CBCs. It was ten days since my last chemo infusion and I was in my nadir, as evidenced by my CBC results. Apparently my numbers were so low that I was to be admitted to the hospital later the same day for an inpatient stay. I was confused and didn't understand all the fuss. Why couldn't I just get my transfusions downstairs and call it a day? What if the hospital also lost my medical records?

After arrival at the hospital and the normal registration and intake process, I found my way up to the 2-West cancer floor. My family of nurses was expecting my arrival and my room was ready. It was as though I never left there at all. I was recognized, and my medical records appeared to be intact. Thank you very much.

I brought my duplicated inpatient stay paperwork package, so we again skipped the half-hour of filling out forms. Terry had packed my duffel bag with all the necessities for a stay of undetermined length.

My mediport was accessed with a needle that only seemed to be two sizes larger each time the procedure was performed. It didn't hurt any less the forty-ninth time than it did the very first time, which now seemed a lifetime ago. Blood was drawn right away for CBCs, and an IV bag of something was plugged in and started as well.

When the CBC results were in a short while later, I was told that I would receive two units of blood and a unit of platelets right away. I guess my fluids were really low. They must have sent me here as a precaution, so I would be able to quickly get all of the attention, pharmaceuticals and blood products I might need.

On Tuesday, there were orders for another unit of platelets and an additional two units of blood. The platelets were drained into me quickly, within an hour, and with no resulting issues.

But, after receiving the first unit of blood I began to shiver uncontrollably. The shivering was a reaction to the blood I was given. This had not happened before and I did not take it as a good sign. Was my body rejecting this blood? Had I developed a resistance to all donor blood?

Would it continue, or was it a fluke? What happens if I can't continue to get my fluids topped off? Oh crap, this can't be good.

I was immediately given Levaquin and Clindamycin. These are antibiotics and I wondered why I got both of them at the same time. The past has shown that I might be allergic, or at least experience an abnormal or adverse reaction, to certain antibiotics as evidenced by my initial problem with cefepime. Won't the fact that the two are given together mask which one was causing a problem, should a problem arise? I should have gone to medical school so I could understand the reasoning behind some of these decisions.

Next, I received an additional unit of blood. Let's recap; a unit of platelets, a unit of blood, a reaction to the blood, two antibiotics working, and now another unit of blood transfused. Things didn't look so rosy at the moment, and they were about to get worse.

After the second unit of blood was received, I developed a fever. At the moment my temperature was 102°, which may not sound too bad for most people, but I was always told that a temperature of 100.5° was life-threatening for me because of my impaired immune system. I theoretically cannot develop a temperature higher than that due to the absence of the required white cells.

Somehow I survived and fell asleep after receiving an additional dose of Clindamycin. Overnight vitals checks offered no evidence of improvement.

Wednesday morning dawned, bringing with it needed relief as my fever had subsided sometime after midnight. I received two more units of platelets without incident, and was cleared for a 6:00 p.m. discharge by the IDC doctor. I was given a prescription for Clindamycin to use at home. Thanks a lot; I'm out of here again.

# Chapter 30

Friday morning CBCs were drawn at FCS, followed by a brief examination and meeting with Dr. Rodriguez. All appeared to be as good as could be expected, but I was to remain on guard for fever.

I was instructed continually for months by all of my medical professionals to seek immediate help if I developed a fever with a temperature of 100.5° or greater. In addition, Dr. Rodriguez told me a number of times to call the FCS answering service anytime his office was closed if I had a problem or developed a fever. An oncologist is always on call to respond to just such an emergency.

Later in the day I received a surprising telephone call from someone at the H. Lee Moffitt Cancer Center in Tampa. Apparently my health plan company arranged to pay the costs for a visit to discuss the feasibility of a bone marrow transplant (BMT). Why did this take since April to arrange? I give up. Would a bone marrow transplant still be feasible? Did I need one? I had a lot of questions and no answers.

I was told by the caller from Moffitt that I had an appointment for a Monday morning meeting with a transplant team. I would need to bring all of my medical and imaging records with me. Hmm, it was Friday afternoon, and they expected me to pull these records together by the end of the business day? They have got to be kidding.

I responded that I may be able to collect my records in time for a Tuesday appointment, but Monday was out of the question. I was not sure there was even a prayer to get that done by the close of business on Monday in order to have the records available for a Tuesday meeting. It would take a miracle, but I said I would do my best to make it happen if we could somehow push the meeting back by one day. After a brief session of begging and being put on hold for a while, we made an agreement that Terry and I would be there for a Tuesday morning meeting. I hoped to somehow get my hands on the very large stack of medical records in time.

After a minor panic attack, I began to formulate a plan. I needed to somehow obtain possession of all my medical records in the remaining ten business hours before beginning a 150 mile trip early Tuesday morning. I made my first call to Mary Ann, a clinician specialist I came to know, admire and respect from our frequent contact while I was an inhabitant of 2-West. Her title is "Advanced Oncology Certified Clinical Nurse Specialist" and her business card sports a healthy dose of alphabet soup as a suffix to her name.

Mary Ann often encouraged me to visit the Moffitt Cancer Center to make sure that I was fully aware of all of my options for treatment. I'm not so sure, in retrospect, she would be thrilled with her choice to encourage me after I made my request for her help.

Mary Ann answered her office phone on the first ring; it may well be my lucky day. My plea for her help was met by a kind and thoughtful, "I'll do my best John, but please realize what you ask may well be impossible to do in such a short window of time." This was good news, more than I could ever expect or even hope for. Mary Ann would be in touch as soon as there was any news or progress made. That would probably be Monday, she said.

# Chapter 31

*A test of the emergency broadcast system*

It was time to put the FCS 24/7 around-the-clock emergency service to a live test. It was 1:45 a.m. Saturday morning, and I woke from a sound sleep shivering uncontrollably. I noticed my pillow looked and felt like it was thrown into a bathtub full of water before being retrieved and placed under my head. Since chemotherapy began back in April, I experienced night sweats much of the time. The fact that my pillow was soaked with perspiration was not unusual. The chills and uncontrollable shivering however, were unusual, and indicated the onset of fever.

In a kitchen cabinet, we keep two oral thermometers and a temporal artery (TA) scanner. The temporal artery runs through your forehead. A temperature measurement there will indicate much the same as a rectal temperature, which is generally one degree warmer than an oral or ear canal temperature measurement. Ear temperature measurements were done routinely while in the hospital as a component of the constant vitals measurements. A TA scanner thermometer uses a sensor that is pressed onto your forehead and dragged across the skin over the temporal artery. It displays a temperature reading in a matter of seconds. I prefer the TA scanner to an oral thermometer because of the fast response and accuracy. If a fever is indicated by the TA scanner, I always double-check the result with an oral thermometer, just to be certain. I have never found the TA scanner to be in error, and I would recommend it to anybody. Those who must wage battle with their children to get a good body temperature measurement would really appreciate the convenience of this handy instrument.

Now, let's get back to the emergency. My TA scanner indicated a temperature of 102.5°, and I verified that with an oral thermometer measurement that was similar; displaying 102°. I hesitated to bother anyone at that time of night (actually early morning), but recalled the insistence of my medical providers that action be taken immediately in such a circumstance. To my surprise, the answering service for FCS picked up on the first ring; maybe this was the right thing to do. I described my general problem and was promptly informed to expect a return call from the doctor on call within the next fifteen minutes. I must say that I was impressed by this reaction to my difficulties, and felt comforted and at ease. It was now 2:00 a.m.

When the fifteen minute mark was reached and time continued to march on, I no longer felt comforted and at ease. I told myself someone would call shortly, and I retook my temperature to kill some time. My fever was unchanged and so was the fact that I had not yet received a return call. It was past 2:20 a.m., more than twenty minutes since my original call for help, so I decided to take some Tylenol and call again.

The answering service picked up on the first ring, and the operator seemed surprised that nobody had called me back. He assured me that he would page the on-call doctor again right away.

At 2:45 a.m., 45 minutes after my first call for help, I was still waiting for a response. My temperature had begun to recede (101.5° using the TA scanner), but I was upset that nobody had yet called me back. When I made my final call to the emergency line, the operator seemed put-out by my repeated calls, but informed me that he would retry the page. I was a little shaken, and wondered what would have happened had my fever not continued to ebb.

By 3:15 a.m. my temperature had fallen to just north of 100° and my anxiety lessened in direct proportion to the continuing drop in temperature. At 3:30, with my temperature at a flat 100°, I returned to bed. I vowed that next time I would not seek help that may never come, and that I would proceed directly to the hospital emergency room. As I reflected on the past few hours, it became apparent that, even if I was called back by the on-call oncologist, I probably would have received instructions to go to the emergency room. In retrospect, I'm not even sure what I expected as a response from the emergency phone call. I had better start thinking things through more thoroughly than I had up until then.

When I got out of bed at sunrise, my temperature was back to normal. There was also a message on my answering machine with a time stamp of 4:46 a.m. from an oncologist to call back if they were still needed. The caller was not Dr. Rodriguez, but I made a note to speak with him about my experience. An intended fifteen minute response time had morphed into nearly three hours. The on-call doctor must have been extremely busy with other emergencies, and unavailable to address my problems. I've yet to meet an oncologist who enjoys much leisure time.

# Chapter 32

Monday, when I returned home after an appointment for CBCs at FCS, there was a phone message from Mary Ann at the hospital. I needed to go to a nearby medical office to pick up all of my imaging records that had been loaded onto a CD. Later, I was to pick up all of the hard-copy, printed records from the Medical Records Office at her hospital. Another miracle, thank you Mary Ann; without your divine intervention this would never have been possible.

I don't know how she accomplished that feat in such a short period of time, but I was extremely grateful. That was not the last time Mary Ann intervened on my behalf.

Tuesday morning, Terry and I made the two and one-half hour trip to Tampa. We travelled over the famous Sunshine Skyway Bridge that spans the mouth of Tampa Bay, and really enjoyed the view from atop this engineering marvel. Not really; I have a mild acrophobia and therefore don't like heights. To be completely honest, they scare the crap out of me. This bridge is 430 feet high and 21,654 feet in length. My butt puckered up as we reached the apex, and I compared the feeling to the way I felt during some of my struggles with AML. I thought if we could just get to the other side, I could surely beat this cancer.

A half-hour later, we arrived at the Moffitt Center and found an open parking space almost immediately. That was nearly a miracle, as we did not see another open space during our long-ish walk to the main entrance.

H. Lee Moffitt Cancer Center and Research Institute is a world-renowned teaching hospital located on the Tampa campus of the University of South Florida. When Terry and I approached the main entrance, we were surprised to discover they had a valet parking service that was staffed by students from the University. So much for my finding-a-parking-space prowess; it would probably be raining when we left the building to walk back to our car.

No hospital visit would be complete without scads of registration paperwork, and Moffitt was no exception. They were kind enough on Friday to direct me to the online Patient Portal to fill out the majority of the required forms. They might have just saved another tree, provided nobody felt the need to print out the forms later.

We waited for quite a while past our appointment time before being escorted from the waiting room into a lab area. There, blood was drawn for CBCs. I don't know why everybody had to have their own individual blood test results. There were so many recent reports available (I even brought the last three with me), but it must have been protocol. Who was I to argue with protocol? Besides, most of the blood flowing through my veins was from donors. Gee, what a waste.

Next, we were guided to an empty room to wait for a member of our transplant team to discuss the concept of transplant and the issues involved. A two-person intern team and a transplant nurse arrived and explained in painstaking detail what the transplant process actually was, what to expect before, during and after transplant, and the associated risks. The process took the better part of an hour, and included a risk assessment that sounded pretty grim from where Terry and I sat.

We were told of the GVHD (graft versus host disease) probabilities and risks faced during the initial four-day chemotherapy session that was designed to bring one as close to death as possible before receiving donor marrow. There would be a thirty day inpatient stay and a three month residency somewhere within a ten to fifteen minute drive radius to the Center.

An *allogeneic* transplant involves receiving donor marrow or peripheral stem cells. An *autologous* transplant involves the infusion of your own, previously-collected marrow. The Moffitt Center told us they would perform an allogeneic transplant only, because of the superior statistical success rate. More information on risks of allogeneic bone marrow transplants will follow.

Terry and I were introduced to more people belonging to our team. Included were the lead transplant doctor, a team of nurses and a social worker who would help us find local housing. They were all very nice, extremely polite and seemed quite adept at all the assigned tasks within their own specialty. Their experience and expertise could never be called into question.

The first task would be to find a suitable donor for bone marrow. A sibling with an HLA match of 10/10 would be best, followed by a sibling HLA match of 8/10. HLA is an acronym for Human Leukocyte Antigen, and is a DNA typing method used to match patients with donors for bone marrow or cord blood transplants. A close or perfect match between patient and donor HLA markers can reduce the risk of GVHD and immune system rejection by the patient. The science of this is quite amazing and a plethora of information can be found at the website for the National Marrow Donor Program[5].

Terry and I were troubled by a statement made by the lead transplant doctor. He used the phrase "Too bad you weren't here before you started chemotherapy. . ." more than once. We questioned why he repeated this, but we never received a direct answer or appropriate explanation.

That was not a good sign. I explained the red tape we tried to unravel back in April *before* chemo was started. We wanted to have this consultation to help determine the correct path to take, but could not afford the asking price. We needed a great deal of help from our insurance company, but Moffitt was out of network, and we were out of luck. I opted to put my life in the hands of Dr. Rodriguez way back then. Now, we were being told that, yes, I should absolutely undergo a bone marrow transplant, regardless of having gone through a chemotherapy regimen plus two complete consolidations.

We asked a lot of questions that were promptly addressed, and took our notes on the fly. The transplant team told us that I should complete my remaining two consolidation chemotherapy sessions, then go directly to

_____

[5] See Appendix A

transplant. We were confused. If a transplant was to be performed, and it would have been better to do it before chemotherapy, why would I continue to receive additional chemotherapy consolidations before moving on towards transplant? I was already in remission. I was also in a very confused state of mind. It dawned on me sometime later that maybe I simply never asked the right questions.

After lunch in the university cafeteria, we had the opportunity to address a few remaining issues in a follow-up meeting. All in all, this was an interesting and informative trip. I was pleased we finally got the opportunity; it might just save my life.

Back at home Tuesday evening, Terry and I discussed the meetings in great detail and referred to our pile of notes taken during our day in Tampa. There were many unanswered questions, and we attempted to put them in some sense of order so each concern would be discussed in context. In addition, I needed to call my extended family to advise everyone that I may go to transplant in a few months, after my final consolidation chemotherapy.

# Chapter 33

When I made the necessary telephone calls to my family, everyone wanted to know what they might do to help. My son and two of my sisters immediately offered to donate the marrow required for the transplant. Because of genetics, my son would not be a suitable donor, but my sisters might be. My oldest sister Patricia has children and would be a less perfect donor given an identical HLA match than Jeanne, who is younger and has no children, except for her rescued dogs. Each offered to be tested right away to find out if they might be a good HLA match. I was humbled by their generosity and told them that a test kit would be sent from Moffitt within the next day or two.

It turned out that Jeanne was already a member of the bone marrow donor registry. Because of her willingness to help others no matter the cost to her, I must put in a shameless plug for an organization she supports. She takes rescued dogs into her home, while searching for a new owner and permanent residence for them. Jeanne often houses four or more of these animals at the same time. The dogs are usually very old, very sick, very abused or a combination thereof. If you care about animals, this organization deserves your support; contact information for New England Paws is included in Appendix A.

Patricia, as I would later discover, was scared to death by just the thought of becoming a bone marrow donor. That was not something she had ever considered, but she was willing to try to save my life. I am truly blessed. If the shoe is on the other foot someday, I'll be the first in line for any of my sisters.

During the next few weeks, I immersed myself in the study of bone marrow/cord blood/stem cell transplants. Adding this new information to the data we collected at Moffitt, I attempted to aggregate and somehow process the mountain of facts, data, charts and probabilities.

Terry and I talked at length about the social and financial ramifications. Impacts included becoming Tampa residents for four months or more, effects on Terry's employment, and the fact that Terry would now become an around-the-clock 24/7 caregiver. At our transplant team meetings, nobody was willing to speak directly to the financial ramifications of BMT.

The financial implications of treating cancer are staggering. Quite near the onset of my disease I learned that many families end up bankrupt sometime during or soon after treatment. It is a shame that someone with a life-threatening disease such as cancer must not only fight for their very survival, but may lose all they have worked for in the prior years of a lifetime.

# Chapter 34

CBCs at FCS Wednesday and Friday showed some recovery of my immune system as indicated by my blood counts. The next Monday, Dr. Rodriguez gave the go-ahead for me to have a tooth extracted as requested by the transplant team at Moffitt. If I went forward with a transplant, they did not want the tooth to generate an infection at the exact time my immune system was least able to defend against it.

Wednesday, after CBCs demonstrated a sustained improvement of my immune system, I visited my dentist for the extraction. He was young and fairly new to private practice. Oh, and he was horrified that I was in the middle of chemotherapy treatments and had a weakened immune system. He also knew that I might never stop bleeding once the fun began.

The young dentist called Dr. Rodriguez to discuss his concerns. I don't know exactly what

Dr. Rodriguez told him, but he instantly appeared more confident and made short work of the extraction after consulting some X-rays taken when I first arrived.

Thursday, the dentist called my home to make sure there were no issues resulting from the extraction. I told him the bleeding had stopped as expected Wednesday afternoon, and all was well. I was surprised to get that phone call; he'll certainly be my dentist of choice for a long time.

Friday brought another round of CBCs. My numbers were holding and the surface area where my molar used to be had already begun to heal. "Great!" said Dr. Rodriguez, "It's time for consolidation #3." Arrangements were made for a Monday arrival for another inpatient stay. This was really getting old and I looked forward to the end of these treatments.

Five days of high dose chemotherapy consolidation #3 passed without any notable issues. Registration through discharge; everything proceeded as planned. I was used to all of it, and the hospital staff was at their best once again. Even the self-administered injection of Neulasta on Saturday was without drama. We were on a roll.

CBCs on Monday, Wednesday and Friday the following week at FCS showed a slow and steady deterioration of my immune system.

Hemoglobin and platelet counts were bordering the danger zone, but I would not receive a fill-up of either. Dr. Rodriguez was worried that I would build up a resistance to donated blood products, and therefore, he would only authorize their use if deemed absolutely necessary. He kept me alive and in remission up to this point, so I trusted his judgment. I felt OK, and even decided to join up with my old golf group for a Sunday game.

# Chapter 35

I gave bone marrow transplant a great deal of thought and consideration before I decided that a transplant was not the right choice for me. That was a decision not made lightly, and one that might even lead to my death.

Terry told me she would honor whatever decision I made, and would support me no matter the physical, emotional or financial cost. The choice was correct, I believe, for both of us.

I will share a few of the reasons that mattered most to me, and helped lead to my choice:

1. Following BMT; no contact for six months with anyone who received a live-virus vaccine (tetanus, chicken pox, measles, diphtheria, polio, influenza, etc.). This no-contact list would include my grandson.

2. No pets (germs, bacteria), no soil or fertilizers (chemicals, mold), no remodel

or construction work (mold, fungus), no golfing (see fertilizers), no swimming or spa (chemicals, bacteria), no bug spray (chemicals) and no live plants (soil, fertilizer). No exposure to the sun for a sixty day minimum, and only then while using skin coverings like hat, gloves, long sleeved shirt, long pants, and showering in SPF-30 sunscreen. This may be OK up north, but I live in Florida.

3. GVHD; graft versus host disease and marrow rejection. This was a large factor in my decision.

4. Common reactions to immunotherapy steroids and drugs used post-transplant to boost the immune system; such as kidney problems, blood sugar issues, magnesium and potassium level issues, tremors, headaches, low blood counts, nausea, diarrhea, G.I. bleeding, darkening patches of skin, edema in legs, feet and arms, cholesterol and triglyceride level issues, joint pain, neuropathy, shortness of breath, weight gain, sleeping problems, osteoporosis, bone necrosis (necessitating joint replacements or plates and pins to hold them together).

The following chart[6] closely fit my situation, and speaks for itself:

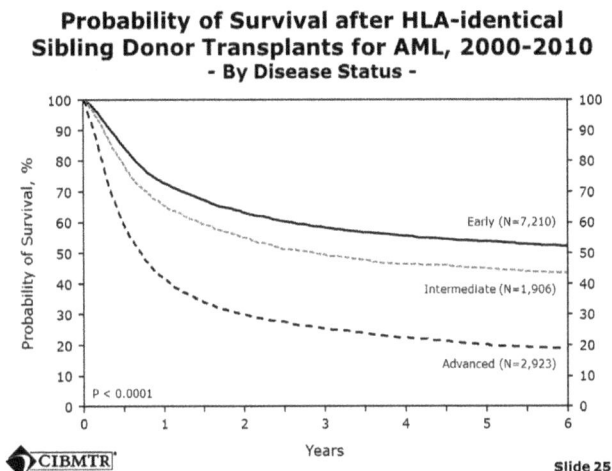

**Probability of Survival after HLA-identical Sibling Donor Transplants for AML, 2000-2010**
- By Disease Status -

If you find yourself in this situation, please conduct your own thorough research, explore all of your options, and do what is right for you, and not what others think is right for you.

Remember, this is *my list*, *my reasons*, and may not apply to anyone other than me. I chose quality versus quantity because I was willing to trade the *hope* of longevity for a *certain*

---

[6] Pasquini MC, Wang Z. Current use and outcome of hematopoietic stem cell transplantation: CIBMTR Summary Slides, 2012. Available at: http://www.cibmtr.org

improvement in quality of life. Take responsibility for your own choices. I made my decision and hold my head high, knowing I must assume full responsibility for any consequences. Make your own decision carefully; things don't always work out the way we plan, do they?

# Chapter 36

It was a beautiful late-August Sunday morning. I enjoyed a cup of coffee before leaving for the short ride to a nearby golf course. I thought of how much I missed being active and outside enjoying the climate here; especially when surrounded by friends.

After drinking my coffee and getting ready to leave the house, I noticed the iron taste of blood in my mouth. The area of my recent tooth extraction was bleeding. The smooth, healing skin that yesterday stretched over the valley where my tooth used to be no longer felt smooth and taut to my tongue. It felt rough, like a patch of window screen had been glued on.

I knew the bleeding was not a good sign, but I was really looking forward to this golf game. I decided to cover the extraction site with sterile gauze that would surely stem the bleeding, and get on with my day. Terry wished me luck as I headed out the door.

During a warm-up on the driving range prior to our round, I started to feel cold. This seemed odd since the temperature was hovering just north of 90°, but I wrote it off as a minor bump in the already rocky road of my recovery. My cart partner noticed I was shivering and asked if I was OK. "Sure," I replied, "just a little chill." He was concerned and wondered whether I should drop out. My goal to fully enjoy that day remained my top priority.

I found that my constant shivering did little to complement my already-shaky golf game. My mouth continued to bleed, and I continued to change out blood-soaked gauze for some new patches I brought with me. The only thing really bothering me was my lack of distance off the tee.

Around the 16th hole, I noticed the shivering was getting worse, and I still couldn't stop the bleeding in my mouth. I finally made the decision to sit out 16, and hoped I could still play holes 17 and 18. Looking back, I'm not sure what I was thinking, but it seemed reasonable at the time. I told my partners that I would be OK when they appeared more concerned. It was thoughtful of them to say that we should just get out of there, but I refused to be the sole cause of ending the round prematurely.

Cancer. Oh, Crap.

We packed our clubs away in my SUV and waited for the other teams to finish. I started to feel a bit worse. The look of me shivering in 95° heat along with a cheek full of bloodied gauze was finally too much for my playing partners to bear. They announced that we were leaving right away. One emphatically stated that I wouldn't be driving us home. But, like a drunk at 2:00 a.m. with a snootful of liquor, I insisted that I could still operate a motor vehicle even though I couldn't finish my round of golf. I realized my reflexes might actually have been impaired when I saw that another one of my group had snatched away my keys and was headed for the driver's seat. I finally surrendered, and hopped into a rear seat to be chauffeured home. I was not a happy camper.

I honestly can't remember if I thanked these friends for making sure I arrived home in one piece, but guys; thank you. Better late than never, I guess.

When I was dropped off at home, Terry took one look at me and reached for the temporal artery scanner. A quick swipe across my forehead and I got the look a mother would give her 6-year-old who just finished playing outside in the snow and somehow misplaced his hat, mittens and boots. She was not pleased, and immediately stormed off to start packing my belongings for a trip to the hospital ER. That's when I took notice of the temperature display; even I was surprised that it read 105°. We knew by now, it was impossible for an impaired immune system such as mine to conjure up a body temperature so high, but there it was.

We also knew enough to skip the call to the emergency hotline and to proceed directly to the hospital. I was quite sure the temperature display of 105° could not have been correct, although I was quite uncomfortable, and shivering and shaking uncontrollably.

# Chapter 37

The ER staff at Lee Memorial Hospital is efficient, kind and competent. In short order, I was in a trauma room being attended to by a nurse. She just offered that condescending grin that nurses are so prone to do when Terry told her what my temperature read back at home; she obviously did not believe it. The grin quickly disappeared when she read the display on the ear canal thermometer she had just used to take my temperature. She looked at it in disbelief, and placed the device on a table before leaving the room. Terry noticed the display that read 105°, and we just smiled at each other.

The nurse reappeared moments later with a replacement for the obviously defective thermometer. When the replacement device also read 105°, we were finally on the same page.

Tubes of blood were taken for CBCs and cross-typing for blood replenishment I was sure to need. We were informed that units of blood and platelets were on the way and we'd get started with infusions ASAP. The port inserted in my wrist vein to draw CBC test-blood was taped in place so it wouldn't move while an IV drip was prepared. A sheet and blanket were thoughtfully put over me in an attempt to lessen the chills I was experiencing.

The nurse hung the clear IV bag on a stand before she pulled back the sheets to gain access to the port in my wrist. Terry's face turned stark white as she was obviously horrified at the sight of something, and she turned away with a shaky hand covering her mouth.

Blood was leaking out of my wrist port onto the bed sheet under the covers where no one would notice. It looked like a quart of the bright red fluid had spilled and pooled beside me. There was a small, red river running from there on the sheet and flowing towards my knees. Crap, that couldn't be good.

The nurse quickly capped off the port and took immediate control of the situation. Bed sheets were whisked away, my blood-soaked clothes removed and put into a plastic bag, and voila; before you could say "exsanguinate," everything was under control. New sheets and a hospital gown for the patient were all in place. Terry still looked like she saw a ghost, and excused herself to visit the restroom in order to vomit in private. She is petrified at the sight of blood to begin with, and seeing my blood spilled like that was too much for her to handle physically and emotionally.

Soon, units of blood and platelets arrived. While my mediport was being accessed with the standard sword-length needles by one nurse, another was hanging the blood and platelet containers on the IV stand. Before beginning the transfusions, they engaged in the familiar duet of name, medical record number, date of birth, etc. I was appreciative of the fact that this formality was never skipped or abbreviated in any way. It spoke well of the infrastructure, training, and attention to detail at this hospital. I wouldn't cry over a little spilled blood. Stuff happens.

Shortly after beginning the transfusions, there was a room reserved for me. We were informed that the 2-West cancer floor was closed for renovations and I would be delivered to the sixth floor. The sixth floor cancer wing housed people who were to have, or were recovering from, a surgery. I was not happy about that because I was accustomed to the second floor nurses, support staff, and the rhythms of the floor and all of its idiosyncrasies. I didn't know what to expect on 6-North, where I was headed.

I was assigned to a private room that was much like a room on 2-West. The nurses and staff were all strangers to me though, and I didn't trust anybody yet. I missed my 2-West nurses, and felt like a schoolboy whose date didn't show for the prom. I don't care how good the treatment of patients was up on 6-North, I wanted my angels back.

Speaking of angels, one of my night shift nurses from 2-West must have drawn the short straw and was caring for me that evening. I had a lot of pain in my pelvis and hips. I didn't know what was causing the pain, but Tylenol was not doing the job of relieving it. I often had bone pain, but it was usually the result of a Neupogen injection that had stimulated an explosive growth of white cells within my bone marrow.

Whenever I sought relief from pain, the standard response from a doctor or nurse was the question: "On a scale of one to ten, with ten representing the worse pain imaginable, what number is your pain?" I always have answered truthfully, and usually any pain was not higher than a five on that scale. That night my pain was at least an eight and the result was that I could not get comfortable enough to sleep. I requested a Demerol injection to ease the pain.

Demerol is used to treat moderate to severe pain. It acts on certain centers in the brain to provide pain relief, and is a narcotic pain reliever similar to morphine.

My nurse returned a short while later with a syringe and announced, "I have good news and bad news." "Great," I said out loud, "half a million comedians out of work and my nurse wants to be funny."

Undaunted by my rude interruption, she continued, "First the bad news; Demerol is no longer on your list of allowed medications," and, after a short pause for effect, "The good news is that something called Dilaudid *is* on your list."

I was informed that Dilaudid is an addictive narcotic that would probably dispatch my pain quickly. I was also told that Dilaudid is much more potent than morphine or Demerol. I was skeptical, but I needed to ease the pain. "Let's do it," I responded without hesitation.

The syringe was emptied slowly, directly into my bloodstream via the mediport. When the first drop of the drug entered my port I was immediately at ease, and swallowed by a warm feeling that is difficult to describe. The feeling of warmth began at the very top of my head and traveled slowly towards my feet, erasing every last bit of pain as it passed. Moments later, I was soundly asleep. I discovered a new favorite, and I completely understood why Dilaudid is classified as an addictive substance.

# Chapter 38

*Waterboarding, anyone?*

My medical team discovered that bacteria invaded my system, probably through the small canyon where my molar used to be. I endured what seemed an endless array of tests, and days filled with X-rays, CT scans and MRIs. I thought I'd seen it all, until I was scheduled for a bronch, which is doctor-speak for bronchoscopy.

After being brought by transport bed to somewhere in the bowels of the hospital, I found myself in a darkened room where I was greeted by a doctor. I would later think of that doctor as the good Dr. Frankenstein.

He explained that the bronch would be a relatively quick procedure that attempts to discover whether or not bacteria are present in the walls of my lungs. "All we need to do is to put a camera into your nasal passage, down your throat and right into your lungs."

"Holy crap," I thought, "Is that all?"

The doctor informed me that he would squirt a numbing fluid into each of my nostrils. He explained, "This may be a little uncomfortable, and may cause you to experience a slight drowning sensation. It's very important that you inhale as much of this fluid as possible."

After that, I would be given goofy juice and he would take care of the rest. He gave me an odd look when I asked for Dilaudid, so I decided not to press it.

A "slight drowning sensation" was a gross understatement. From point-blank range, the doctor squirted the contents of a tube directly into one nostril and I instantly felt that I might drown. I couldn't breathe because my gag reflex kicked in to make sure that drowning was avoided. "Good job," he said, "now for just one more," you know, as if I had somehow forgotten that I had two nostrils.

The other nostril was squirted before I had time to react, and I breathed in deeply through my nose in a heroic attempt to get it over with. The drowning sensation became worse with the increase of fluid volume running down my airway. I already felt the numbing sensation taking hold. It felt like my insides turned to stone.

The last thing I remember was a mask being placed over my nose and mouth. Upon waking up in the recovery room I was groggy, and felt like a camcorder was somehow pushed through my nose and down my throat; but only because that was pretty much what took place.

Results from my waterboarding were inconclusive. I was deemed not well enough to be subjected to further testing for bacteria; so they came up with a better idea. They wanted me to have intravenous penicillin around the clock, just in case the bacteria had somehow escaped and found a place to hide within my heart. Liquid penicillin would be infused intravenously 24/7 for the next three-to-four weeks.

My choices were two:

1). Remain in the hospital hooked up to a regular IV, or;

2). Get a fanny pack-mounted, miniature portable pump hooked up and routed to my mediport. I would need to return to the hospital every day for a refill of the penicillin and an operational check of the pump.

Those were some choices, huh? I elected to get the heck out of there, even if it meant I would be sporting the latest in metro-male fanny packs for the next month or so.

I was sent over to the IV Center offices to be fitted and plumbed for the latest in portable medical pump apparatus. A small digitally-

Cancer. Oh, Crap.

controlled pump with a clear plastic bag of penicillin and a length of tubing were attached to my port and placed in a black fanny pack. The tubing was routed under my shirt and directly to my chest mediport. The pump was programmed and checked for operation and fitted with a new 9V battery. It was set to run for 24 hours, at which time the penicillin container bag should be empty. As I later discovered, there was an annoying alarm that would sound continuously once the penicillin was depleted, or if somehow the flow to my port ceased for any reason. Not to worry, I would figure out how to silence the alarm when necessary.

I was now able to be discharged, and I would keep pushing until all of the required signatures were collected and I could hit the road. It was a long and exciting week, but I was ready to get back home as soon as possible. Terry was working that day because we weren't sure of my status, so I called on my friend John Lee for a ride home.

# Chapter 39

Monday, September 5$^{th}$ was Labor Day. We'd been at this almost five months now, including initial chemotherapy and three consolidations. I won't lie to you; I was tired and still didn't know what tomorrow would bring. I remained in complete remission, but was looking at daily visits to the hospital to have a refill of fanny pack-penicillin. When the month was over, I had another consolidation to look forward to.

My daily visits to the IV Center passed uneventfully. I normally arrived fifteen minutes early for my 1:00 p.m. standing appointment and I received attention immediately, despite the fact I arrived during the lunch hour.

In the middle of September, friends John and Robin from Massachusetts arranged to come by for a short visit. They made the trip to see us from their second home in Lakeland, Florida. John was the best man at my wedding, and although we don't often visit each other or even talk on the telephone regularly, it is always great to see him and Robin. Ours is a low-key friendship that will last a lifetime in spite of the distance and circumstance that keep us geographically separated. Terry and I were really glad that John and Robin chose to visit.

Wednesday, September 28th was the last day of my penicillin and fanny pack. It had been a very long 24 days that I was happy to see only in the rear view mirror. My mediport was flushed, as it had been every day, and the tubing and needle inputs were removed. A large rectangular bandage was put into place over the skin covering my port, and I was on my way.

I went to FCS on Mondays, Wednesdays and Fridays to have CBCs drawn. My numbers were stable and improving, and I felt generally very well. On Friday, October 7, Dr. Rodriguez announced that my fourth and final consolidation would begin on Monday, October 10th.

I proposed to Dr. Rodriguez that my admittance date be delayed by two days. Past experience indicated that the timing of a Monday start would put my nadir period onto a weekend as it had in the past. Transfusions, if needed, would not be available because of this timing issue. I did not want to end up in the ER on a Sunday afternoon again.

Dr. Rodriguez understood my logic, and I was scheduled to be admitted for consolidation #4 on Wednesday, October 12th.

Consolidation #4 that began on Wednesday was completed without incident, and I was discharged the following Monday, October 17th. I loved it when a plan came together. If history offered an accurate indication, I should be feeling well right through the following weekend, then crash sometime on a weekday. We'll know by the Monday morning CBCs if transfusions are needed, and, if so, get them ASAP *before* I crash. Catastrophe avoided. Logic prevailed.

We were soon to discover that I was very, very wrong.

CBCs drawn on Wednesday indicated blood counts that were slowly slipping towards dangerous territory, and we voiced hope that they held in the safe zone, if only through the next weekend as planned.

Friday morning, my CBCs revealed a more disturbing path towards trouble, but the test results were not bad enough to warrant a blood or platelet transfusion. Dr. Rodriguez patiently explained that my body was building up a tolerance to platelets and other blood products, so it was not wise to get them until, and unless, absolutely necessary. I knew the trending tendencies of my blood count characteristics well enough to predict that I would crash sometime within the next few days. The transfusion center down one floor was not open on Sundays, so I attempted to negotiate an alternative. No dice; we would just hope for the best. It seemed as though I outsmarted only myself with the change in admission dates, and now I was praying to get through the weekend unscathed by any major event.

# Chapter 40

It is a glorious Sunday around noon in mid-October. The sun is streaming in through the sliding glass doors, silently massaging my back as I sit at the kitchen table eating a sandwich while navigating the large weekend newspaper. A family of ducks at lake's edge just outside my door quacks out an opera only they know the lyrics to, and there is a large snow-white egret looking for his lunch. My northern friends refer to this place as 'God's Waiting Room', while the automobile license tags sport oversized oranges and proclaim this to be the 'Sunshine State'.

After lunch, I headed for the living room to watch a game on television. It's been a long time since I've felt this well and Terry seems pleased that the worst appears to be over. She has put her recent memories into an imaginary drawer labeled *"History – let's hope the worst has passed."*

Not five minutes later, an all too familiar feeling washes over me and I instinctively know what the next few hours will bring; not because I'm smart, but rather because we've been through this before. A quick swipe over my forehead with the temporal artery scanner reveals an elevated temperature of 102.9°. I try to head this fever off at the pass by swallowing a few Tylenol pills. Ten minutes later my temperature is somewhere north of 103° and I confirm this finding with an oral thermometer. My system is obviously trying to fight off an infection of some kind.

Terry is already packing my overnight bag for a trip to the emergency room. There is no point in calling my oncologist's answering service because we know the drill. Get to the emergency room ASAP. As we leave the house my thermometer displays 104° and I know we're in trouble again.

We arrived at the ER within 15 or 20 minutes and met with a nurse right away. The usual paperwork was dealt with quickly because we were really good at this by now. My temperature was down to 103° and I was brought to a nearby trauma room where blood was drawn for CBCs. After being dressed in the standard hospital gown, the mediport implant in my chest was accessed and flushed with heparin. I was hooked up to IV fluids and an IV antibiotic to begin fighting whatever it was that invaded and got past my lowered defense shields. Since being discharged from my last round of consolidation chemotherapy a week ago, I remained in a bubble, worried that a rogue infection would seize any opportunity to bring me down. It now appeared that my bubble had sprung a leak.

A unit of irradiated blood arrived at my room in the ER and joined the fluids and antibiotics marching through clear tubing into my mediport. I felt awful and began to vomit uncontrollably into the nearest receptacle that happened to be an empty wastebasket at my bedside. That was new, and didn't bode well for my immediate future. The vomiting subsided within a few minutes, and an ER doctor informed me that I was headed for the ICU. I responded that I didn't belong in the Intensive Care Unit; send me up to the 2-West cancer floor and they'll fix me up. I was afraid that, if sent to the ICU, I would never be allowed to leave. Like the Hotel California; you can check out anytime you like, but you can never leave. Again, it seemed that my negotiating skills abandoned me in my time of need. The doctor was insistent that I needed to be in the ICU, and that was where I was headed. Terry already called the nurses on 2-West to enlist their help in convincing the ER staff that I should be on the cancer floor, also to no avail. It appeared that my next destination was the ICU, and I was not happy.

I arrived at the ICU on a transport bed with an IV hanger and a variety of medicines and fluids. I was ushered into a dark room with a large family of machines humming a sad beeping song accompanied by colorful flashing LEDs. I was assisted from the transport bed onto my new hospital bed. I was really tired and didn't feel well at all. Terry handed me a pan of some sort as she saw I was getting ready to vomit again. Something was really wrong. Throughout my struggle I had been sick before, but not like this. I needed to use a toilet urgently but could not see a bathroom within my new confines. When I asked where the bathroom was located, the nurses just grinned. Oh, thanks anyway, but I don't want a catheter and a bedpan. A urine bottle was brought to me and a portable bedside toilet was wheeled in. "Knock yourself out," they seemed to say, but not out loud. Telemetry sensors were glued to my skin to send signals that would be displayed and recorded somewhere on the wall of instrumentation behind me. I wondered if my ticket had been punched, and it was the end of the road for me. I remember drifting off to sleep while listening to the steady beeping of vitals monitoring equipment.

The next few days are a hazy memory for me. I can never seem to clearly recall any particulars from my time in the ICU. I think it is the brain's way to shield one from the awful truth of what might have been.

A doctor from IDC listened to Terry when she pointed out that I was having an adverse reaction to the vancomycin I was receiving. It was ordered withdrawn immediately and replaced with a substitute. I was later told that was the time my condition began to improve.

The root cause for my visit to the ICU was determined to be E. coli. It had permeated my gut because my platelets were so few. From there, it was all downhill.

I remember that the nurses and aides were kind and considerate, and I remember Terry was at my side. I have vague and fleeting memories of doctors and priests watching over me at various times, performing their own separate rituals. I also have memories of Dr. Rodriguez and Mary Ann looking concerned as they stood over me, and I remember some of my 2-West angels writing a get-well wish on the wall-mounted whiteboard.

How I survived all this, I honestly cannot say for sure. Divine intervention would be my best guess. I may not be worthy, but faith has served me well. I still have the feeling that I was able to outrun the devil by only seconds; just as he was about to grab me by the ankles, I was able to slip away.

I somehow made it through another time of crisis and was pronounced to be well enough on Wednesday, October 26$^{th}$ to take up residence down on 2-West; back to my angels. I was once again a happy camper.

# Epilogue

Room 2338 on floor 2-West was the final hospital room I would inhabit; at least for now. I remain in full remission from leukemia as of this writing, and somehow I survived and lived to tell of my full-on chemotherapy regimen and four additional consolidation chemotherapy sessions, and the nadir crashes that followed.

Following my hospital discharge on November 1st, CBCs at Florida Cancer Specialists were drawn three days per week until my blood counts were stable and improving.

My mediport was removed in May of 2012 in an outpatient surgery, and I currently return every three months to visit Dr. Rodriguez and have CBCs done; stat!

I will remember each individual involved in every aspect of my care throughout my journey; each day I silently offer a sincere "thank you" to all. If it were not for you, I may not be here to tell this story with a decidedly happy ending.

I often reflect upon what have I learned from my experience with leukemia. First and foremost, I credit a positive attitude for my success. I was not always bright and chipper, and often did not feel well, but I did always believe that I could and would beat this disease, and woke up every day ready to do battle. Hope springs eternal.

I learned to be a participant in my care, not an onlooker. I learned to be persistent; to expect the best and prepare for the worst. Don't take *no* for an answer. Do your own research. I learned to ask questions at each and every step, and learned that I deserve a response and a reason for any contemplated procedure.

I learned that those who choose to care for cancer patients are a special breed. They witness the horror and tragedies heaped upon others and somehow get up each morning to continue the fight. Their compassion for others comes from a bottomless well. Take the time to find out about your caregivers. Ask questions and know their name and their story; they each have a reason for doing what they do. Everyone is touched by cancer in some way, whether a loved one in their immediate family, a relative, a friend or neighbor. As a very wise man once said,

*"No one fights alone."*

John J. Powers III

None of us know how long we'll be here; enjoy the time you have today and revel in your journey through life.

*Special thanks to Patricia Gorman for her role as copy editor, medical-reference consultant and sounding board.*

# Appendix A

*Where to turn for help and education,*
*And where your help is needed.*

The Leukemia & Lymphoma Society
http://www.lls.org/
> National Marrow Donor Program  BE THE MATCH ®
> http://marrow.org/

The American Red Cross
http://www.redcross.org
> National Institutes of Health
> http://www.nih.gov

National Cancer Institute
http://www.cancer.gov
> American Society of Clinical Oncology
> http://www.cancer.net/

Center for International Blood and Marrow Transplant
Research
http://www.cibmtr.org
> WebMD
> http://www.webmd.com/


*And for our canine friends that need your help:*

PAWS New England
http://www.pawsnewengland.com

www.ingramcontent.com/pod-product-compliance
Lightning Source LLC
Chambersburg PA
CBHW050121280326
41933CB00010B/1194